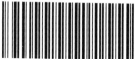

WHISPERS IN THE PEWS

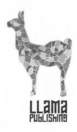

Disclaimer: The information in this book is based on the opinions, knowledge, and experience of the authors. The authors will not be held liable for the use or misuse of the information contained herein.

Publishing and Design Services: MartinPublishingServices.com

ISBN: 978-1-7327335-0-3 (paperback), 978-1-7327335-1-0 (epub)

Morris, Chris (2018-11-16). Whispers in the Pews: Voices on Mental Illness in the Church.

WHISPERS
IN THE PEWS

Voices On Mental Illness
In The Church

EDITED BY CHRIS MORRIS

LLAMA
PUBLISHING

ADVANCE PRAISE FOR
WHISPERS IN THE PEWS

"I am ridiculously excited for the stories in this book to be shared. There is an incredible need to discuss the reality of mental illness and how the church can improve how it addresses this."

—Colleen English, Founder of Rettland Foundation

"I cannot imagine Jesus scolding someone with a mental illness, telling them to just get over it, try harder, memorize more verses. No, He would listen. He would love. He would be filled with compassion. And even He was deemed mentally ill in his time, his miracles attributed to demonic activity. In short, Jesus empathizes with people who don't fit a culture's mold. But the church? We can either cause more suffering or create pathways of hope. Sadly, through ignorance and Christian platitudes we've done more of the former than the latter. This book offers incredibly precious insight to help the church become like Jesus for those who suffer. Read this book. Give it to your pastors and leaders. Revolutionary seems too small a word."

—Mary DeMuth, author of *The Seven Deadly Friendships*

"Compassion is the antidote to stigma, and it only begins when we hear the stories of real men and women who suffer from mental illness. Chris Morris is doing the church a tremendous service with this book. It should be required reading for anyone who considers himself or herself to be a follower of Jesus."

—David Edward Cummings, PhD,
Professor of Microbiology, Point Loma Nazarene University,
Host of the SoulCare Podcast, Elder at
Pathways Community Church, Santee, CA

"Chris Morris has compiled honest and raw stories that give sight into the heart of many Christians who have battled, or are battling, mental illness. *Whispers in the Pews* brings to light that mental health matters and how it hasn't always mattered in the Christian community, and it needs to. Our churches need to be a place where all are welcome, no matter one's story. Chris has written a thought-provoking book that will stir up your heart to be a part of the change we need to see."

—Shawn Elizabeth George,
Inspirational Author, Writer, and Speaker

"Finally, someone is speaking out on a deep and important issue that simply does not get talked about enough in our faith communities. Thank you, Chris, for your honesty and bravery. May these words move us all to deeper and more compassionate action."

—Jeff Goins, bestselling author of *The Art of Work*

CONTENTS

WHY I CREATED THIS BOOK

The statistics surrounding mental health are alarming, and it's no exaggeration to say mental illnesses are nearly epidemic in scope. Except even the use of the word *epidemic* is problematic in the mental illness community. Epidemics describe outbreaks of contagious diseases like malaria or swine flu. Nobody is going to catch PTSD by sharing the same airspace with someone who is afflicted.

No matter what word we use to describe the crisis, diagnosed mental illnesses are on the rise. Studies show that as many as one in four people in the United States are diagnosed with a mental illness. And these statistics don't include those who have not sought treatment or diagnosis.

Bottom line—mental illness isn't going away any time soon. And yet, the church at large has had a mixed response to mental illnesses. The church should be the one place where people are accepted as they are, no matter the details. Jesus accepted everyone who came across his path—adulterers, tax collectors, fishermen, critics. It didn't matter. As His footprint upon the earth, the church should be the same.

Even with, or perhaps especially with, mental health conditions, the instinct should be to lean into kindness and love. The local church body should gather around, provide a place of safety and transparency, upholding those who are not well in their midst.

And this is exactly what happens—sometimes. There are pastors who are actively looking to normalize mental health conditions by mentioning depression alongside diabetes as an illness that can be treated.

But for every pastor looking to build a healthy understanding of mental illnesses, there is a pastor lumping depression in with pornography, equating anxiety with faithlessness, telling their congregation to avoid medicine for treatment, or otherwise refusing to recognize the complexity of mental illnesses.

And mental health conditions are complex. Certainly there is often a spiritual element, in no large part because of the thoughts that bombard those of us with mental illnesses. But there's usually more going on aside from the spiritual.

There are spiritual disciplines that can help those suffering from depression, but often it's not enough. And yes, talking with a pastor or a counselor can certainly provide some relief for anxiety, but that's not always the path forward either. Sometimes medicine is the answer, or at least part of the answer. And sometimes, there is no answer. Sometimes, trauma has left an indelible mark upon a person that cannot be overcome on this side of eternity.

Many mental illnesses are caused by severe trauma; more specifically, the body or mind's response to these terrible traumas. Mental illness then is often a function of this busted world that we exist in. Put differently, some percentage of mental illnesses wouldn't exist without the sin that has run rampant in this world. But because the world is broken, people are left to respond to the sin that's been committed against them, often as children before they have developed healthy coping skills.

How can anyone tell the woman who suffers from PTSD as a response to being used in pornography as a three-year-old that she should just suck it up and deal with it, maybe pray a little harder and things will get better? No, her suffering is the result of evil, through and through; she's just trying to deal with the consequences of sin against her in her life.

How can anyone tell the young man who is battling depression because of his abusive upbringing with a violent alcoholic father that a little more Bible reading and some memorization of a few verses will make the nightmares go away? No, that's not how it works.

Recovery from trauma is hard. The mind and body have their own ideas about how to heal. Yes, of course the spirit and soul are also involved in the recovery process, but mind and body are equal parts of the human experience.

That's not to insinuate every mental health condition comes from trauma. But even when the root isn't trauma, there is still complexity involved. Some come from chemical imbalances… and no, that's not a cop-out. This is why antidepressants ease the burden for many suffering from severe depression—because these medications work to balance out various neurotransmitters. This is why some diagnosed as bipolar are able to find rest from the highs and lows with lithium—because a lithium imbalance was the problem in the first place.

Unfortunately, these truths are not always appreciated nor understood in the church at large. Many pastors paint with broad strokes, equating any mental illness with immaturity in the faith. It's uncomfortable at best, and fear-inducing at worst, to tell a pastor that he's wrong. Especially when it's hard to nail down why he's wrong.

Because of this discomfort, many choose to put on a happy, shiny Christian mask and act like they're not hurting. It's more painful to confront church leadership and answer all the accusations and questions.

Even more disheartening than putting a mask on, many with mental illnesses choose to step away from the church altogether. They've been hurt too often, and too consistently, to have any space left in their hearts for trust. So they hang tight to a belief in Jesus, but walk away from the church because it hurts too much. Some of the voices you'll read in this book have walked away from church for this very reason.

Church, we can do better. We must do better.

We have to grapple individually and in the context of community with difficult questions. Does loving someone mean never calling them to account on things that seem wrong? Can we question the legitimacy of a diagnosis if it seems like more might be going on? When it comes to mental health, where is the line between pointing out sin and being presumptuous?

There is no single answer to any of these questions, because there's no single story to follow. No two people have walked the same path that brought them to a mental illness. Yes, this is obvious, but its ramifications are far-reaching. Every person brings their own brand of wounding, their own scent of pain, and their own battles.

This reality is why I've gathered almost two dozen voices to share their stories. It's only in listening—truly listening with every fiber of our being—to story after story of mental illness that we are able to see just how different every person is, even when the diagnosis is the same.

Mental illness isn't a simple diagnosis, under any circumstances. It's not like a fractured shoulder blade, where the path to healing is clear. With a shoulder, the bone needs to be set, the shoulder needs to be immobilized, and healing will take place. If there's a complex fracture, then surgery might be necessary.

But, the basic path is the same. This is never true with mental health conditions. Too often the church has treated those with mental illnesses as though there is a straightforward path toward healthier living, and that's been painful to bear.

Whispers in the Pews has been written because I am convinced stories will be the catalyst for change in the church. By hearing the pain and the victories that others have experienced, my hope is that there will be room for a new way to approach mental health—one that sees the person before the health condition.

My hope is this book will open the eyes of pastors and church leaders by sharing the real-life stories of those who are in the middle of the battle. Some have experienced great hope from their faith communities. Some have experienced horrible things and have walked away from the church. Some have made the choice to remain strong, despite painful words from the pulpit about what it means to be a Christian.

The only common thread through all these stories is mental illness. My prayer is that you will read with an open heart. I pray that you will learn to see the complexity of the mental health world. I pray that you will find your own heart softened toward the plight of those in the mental illness community. I pray that, like my own pastor, you will find the courage to state with no qualms that the church is the best place to come for those who are weary and broken.

SUICIDE FEELS LIKE A DIRTY WORD

BY AARON J. SMITH

Suicide feels like a dirty word. It's as if we of faith can't talk about it or even utter its name. It's something dark and sinister, something evil, something never to be invoked. But it's a reality in this world. People die by suicide. When this happens, questions float to the surface of our churches.

Will suicide send you to hell?

How could anyone be so selfish?

What does the Bible say about it?

I once watched a pastor—indeed, a whole church—field, wrestle, and attempt to answer these questions after suicide claimed the life of a prominent member of the congregation. There were prayer meetings, a Sunday morning dedicated to talking about what happened, and countless phone calls among the people of the pews.

With time and distance from the tragedy, rumors started to spread. Some people were devastated by the rumors. Other people moved on with their lives. Within a year, the suicide of this man, who was once an elder of the church, was nothing more than a sad memory slowly fading out in the life of the church. There was no further talk about it. I mean, what else can people say?

But there is so much more to say about suicide, about self-harm, about addiction, about mental illness.

In my early twenties, I thought I might have a mental illness. Turns out I was right—I was diagnosed bipolar II when I was twenty-eight. As I was learning about the illness, I came across something interesting: excessive guilt is one of the symptoms of the disease. I mentioned this to my pastor, and he was genuinely surprised. He had no direction or guidance for me, but stayed in this stunned state.

Can't blame him. After all, I had grown up hearing that guilt was a tool the Holy Ghost used to call us to repentance. That creates a paradigm where everything fits nicely together—the hand of God used guilt for our correction and edification. Now, suddenly, I was learning that excessive guilt was also a symptom of a sickness of the mind.

Things got gray for me after that. It wasn't all clear-cut and easy to define. I was facing the maybe-reality that the guilt I had associated with sin could be nothing more than a misfiring of my neurons.

And my pastor was surprised at it. The spiritual leader to whom I looked for guidance, teaching, and wisdom didn't have a healthy paradigm for mental illness. Over the last few years, I've learned that he's not the only spiritual leader without a paradigm for people like me—those in the mental illness community.

We see it all the time in tweets, quips, and Facebook posts from Christians:

Depression is just not being immersed enough in the Bible.

Anxiety can be beaten by fixing our eyes on God.

Mental illness is simply the result of not loving Jesus enough or not reading the Bible enough or not praying enough.

Even the way we pit "secular" counseling against "biblical" counseling reveals our true colors. As Christians, we don't know how to think cohesively about mental illness. We reduce mental illness to bad feelings that a person just needs to get over. There is no room for biochemical imbalances or trauma-induced states.

There's no concept of medicine as a tool of healing. Mental illness has no real place, so it's lumped together with sin and treated not as an illness but as a flaw.

Even though the Bible is filled to overflowing with people who clearly suffered from mental illnesses, the Bible doesn't directly talk about mental illness. We are so afraid of things that don't fit in our neat little compartments that we refuse to take into consideration the fact that psychosis, addiction, and suicidal ideation are actual things, and not somehow caused by demonic influence in a person's life.

Instead we make up pop theology to rely on rather than be "corrupted" by secular psychologists. We are quick to ignore the fact that mental illnesses all too often lead to suicide and tragedy. Because we don't have the words to talk about those with mental illnesses or the frame of reference to think about them, we often find ourselves without compassion to suffer with them.

Isn't suffering with your neighbor—compassion—the embodiment of loving them as you would love yourself?

Imagine you were thrust into this world of mental illness, diagnosis after diagnosis thrown at you, trying to find something that sticks. Clinical depression. Generalized Anxiety Disorder. OCD. PTSD. Bipolar. Schizophrenia. It's enough to make your head spin. This was precisely my experience as a young adult.

I took this brand-new set of diagnoses to church and asked people who said they loved me to help support me as I figured everything out—meds, treatment, counseling, and just learning what it means to live with mental illness. Instead of tenderness and compassion, my fresh hurt was responded to with, "You just need to pray more and have more faith."

The answer sounds so certain, as if they had attended medical school, had a master's in counseling, and had come up with a better solution to mental illness than the countless other counselors and doctors out there. It's not love to take someone's complex illness and pretend there is a simple answer to it. But that was my experience, and the experience of so many others.

Trite talk like this is hurtful at best, dangerous at worst, because of the nature of mental illnesses. Almost all mental illnesses include feelings of deep worthlessness that pierce our minds uninvited and get deep into our hearts. We begin to believe these cognitive distortions about ourselves. We begin to believe we can't do anything right. We begin to believe we are wastes of space. We begin to believe the lies about how we are a burden to others. That the world is better off without us, and no one would miss us.

When we dare open up about our illness to people, it's scary. We are becoming vulnerable, showing our deepest wounds. This is our shadow place, the place we keep hidden from outsiders. We are inviting you in to see us at our most naked.

Far too often, the response to our vulnerability is an earnest over-spiritualization of our problem. As if we haven't gnashed our teeth before the Lord, begging for relief. But apparently, we haven't prayed enough, we don't have enough faith, it's our fault we suffer an illness of the heart and mind. Somehow, if we could just pull it together, we could beat this illness, find healing, and not be sick. But that's not how mental illnesses work.

Mental illness is not exclusively for the spiritually weak, because it's not a spiritual problem. It's not something to just get over with prayer, essential oils, or any other magic bullet the church might be peddling. It's a real issue, something wrong with the body, just like diabetes or tuberculosis. And it can be just as deadly. This is why we need to talk about suicide, mental illness, counseling, and psychiatric medicine. These things are real; they exist in the pews we inhabit and the pulpits we listen to.

What would it be like to talk about mental illness in church? Not just at the suicide of a beloved person in the church. Rather to talk about it as a reality of life, because indeed it is. Instead of holding emergency prayer meetings to try and triage the trauma, what if we developed transparency in our congregations that allowed people to be seen as ill and in need of love and support before mental illness brings them to crisis?

You don't have to know what to do—just be present. That's what was missing from the aftermath of the suicide I mentioned earlier. That's what was missing from my pastor's reaction to the symptoms of my mental illness. That is what is often missing in the walls of our church.

Being present is one of the most powerful things that can be done in the face of mental illness. It doesn't entail much more than your physical body being in the same room as the person you are being there for. It's a statement of love and compassion, of caring and acceptance. Being present doesn't have an expiration date either—not when it comes from Jesus's heart and is for those whose lives are being torn to shreds.

After the suicide, the church moved on. But the family didn't. How could they? The heart of their family was ripped out of their chest. For a while, some people would check on them, but after a time, the trickle of people dried up and the family was left alone. No one remained present in their grief. It's as if people assumed that the family had moved on because time had passed.

Grief isn't a linear, timed process, though. It's chaos. It's twisty, curvy, and scrambled up. The closer you get to the tragedy the more tangled the grief web becomes. This twisted, chaotic thing is the aftermath of suicide, the aftermath of a mental illness crisis, the aftermath of a broken brain.

Grief often stalks the mentally ill and the ones close to them. Grief can come to rest on the quiet and the lonely, the broken and tired, the hurt and forsaken.

There is no cure for grief, but there is an easing of the pain. Be present. Mental illness, tragedy, and grief need other people. We need other people. The church has let many of us with mental illness down. When I needed direction and encouragement to seek counseling, I received nothing from the pastor I talked to.

How different my life would have been if I had gotten encouragement to seek professional counseling, if I had been told that it was okay and not some scheme of the devil to lure me into secular thinking? But that's the lie I was raised with. So of course suicide and mental illness became dirty words, only to be whispered or kept to ourselves.

It's the result of something the church refuses to acknowledge as a reality of life in this day and age. Of course there are gossipy whispers, rumors, and judgment swirling in the aftermath of tragedies that could have been prevented within a transparent church. We were never given the go-ahead to talk about it in the open and confront the lies. Of course mental illness was for "those people" and not for us good, strong Christians. So many of us have never been told it's not a spiritual problem.

Those of us with mental illness need other people in our lives because mental illness is an isolating thing. Whether it's the self-isolation that comes with depression or the isolation we feel as people pull away from our times of psychosis, living with mental illness is lonely. We need support systems, people willing to wrestle with the hard questions and maybe intervene in our lives before it becomes too late, before it becomes terminal.

Can the church be a support system? Yes. Will it be a support system? I don't know—I hope so. That's hard to say because I love the church. But my history with mental illness and the church tells me that the church can be a deadly place for people with mental illness. A congregation was willing to talk briefly about suicide when it touched their lives. That's a good thing, but it breaks me that it took a suicide to start the conversation that ended all too quickly.

This is an ongoing conversation we need to have because mental illness is an ongoing reality in the lives of the people we love. Failure to address this adds fuel to the guilt-fires of those in the throes of a mental illness. These are the lies that bind. These are the untruths that keep the captives in chains. These are the words that can kill.

But we are made for freedom. We are made to breathe deep and walk in wellness. Mental illness doesn't get the last say. We have the ability to change the conversation about and around mental illness in the church. We are the agents of freedom. We don't need to have dirty words.

We don't need to fear mental illness or somehow see it as a sign of spiritual sickness. We get to liberate mental illness and those who suffer from the years upon years of guilt, condemnation, and isolation. You and I can do this, together. The mentally sick and the mentally stable, working and walking side by side towards wholeness and freedom. No more calling mental illness sin. No more leaving it to blossom in death. We can change everything.

Things must change. If they stay the same, we are going to have more hurt, more isolation, more suicide in our church bodies. That's not the Jesus way, the way of loving your neighbor as you do yourself.

And who is more your neighbor than the one sitting next to you on Sunday mornings? Love them, care for them, and be there for them. Don't be afraid of hard conversations with some uncomfortable answers. Talk about mental illness. Talk to those of us who have mental illness. Let the conversations come from the pew and the pulpit.

It's time for us to not fear words like suicide, psychosis, and addiction. It's time for us to speak about the reality of depression and anxiety. It's time for mental illness to be as readily talked about as cancer, diabetes, and thyroid problems.

Only when we talk about these things, dragging them into the light, can we truly see the pain, isolation and suffering. Only when we see these things clearly can we begin to be present with compassion. Only with compassion can we love people the way Jesus does. And love leads to healing, to acceptance, to wholeness.

Without wholeness, our fragmented lives will only continue to shatter and splinter, no matter the effort we attempt to put forth. Wholeness is what we need. Wholeness in body, in mind, in heart, in community. How else are we going to respond in love to suicide, mental illness, and physical need? How else but together, whole, are we going to be able to take on the hard task of true compassion, truly showing up, truly loving and providing for those who need it?

In the Corner

by Lindsay A. Franklin

I'm three years old, and I'm alone in a dark corner. I don't know how long it's been since my childcare provider put me there, but I've been watching the sun go down. The corner gets darker.

I look on, puzzled, as my big sister Genny argues with the childcare provider. "Why is Lindsay in the corner? Why is she being punished? Lindsay is never in trouble. Let me talk to my sister!"

But she's not allowed. The childcare provider spares me one sidelong glance, then turns back to Genny. "Your sister is being punished because she was *very* bad. Go play in the other room."

And then I'm utterly alone again. Fear pools in my stomach then spreads all throughout my body. What will my mom say when she comes to pick us up? What will she say when they tell her what I've done? I want to cry, but I can't. I'm numb. I don't understand what has happened, but I know it's all my fault. The grown-up said it was. It must be true.

It's a relief when Mama comes to get me and I discover the childcare provider has told her nothing. That's good. That's good because I don't want to be in trouble anymore. If she hasn't told, I won't tell either. I'm too ashamed of myself to tell, so Mama never has to know.

And I don't tell for thirty years. I don't tell about how the two older boys and one girl pulled me behind a play kitchen at our after-school daycare, stripped off my clothes, and molested me. I don't tell about how one of our childcare providers caught them in the act, then punished me. I never tell because, even after I'm old enough to know better, I drown in shame over how I must have invited their violation. They must have seen something in me, on me, through me that told them I wanted them to violate me in that way. There must have been something inherently perverted and disgusting about me, or else that wouldn't have happened...would it?

And I don't understand until I'm thirty-five years old that I have lived most of my life with PTSD. Being violated and then punished for it is my earliest memory, and it has shaped the deepest parts of who I am, affecting how I view the world around me. A world that, for all its joys and laughter and delight, is also full of darkness and danger and oh so much shame. This is the first lesson life taught me, and I will never escape it.

I have Donald Trump to thank for finally being diagnosed.

Because now it's October 2016, and I'm alone in a dark corner again. This time I've put myself there—the corner of the bathroom, within convenient distance of tissues and the toilet bowl, in case I need to vomit again.

Why am I feeling this way? Why do I suddenly feel like I'm three years old again, alone and afraid and sick? Disgusted and disgusting.

Why am I coming undone at the seams?

The Access Hollywood tape scandal has just broken. Many years prior, Mr. Trump had been recorded as he described in lewd terms putting his hands on women—not asking, just grabbing—and he noted that women allowed him to do this because of the power and influence he wielded. When I first heard the news, I was revolted by that old conversation. I was grieved for any potential victims, if Mr. Trump did indeed behave in the way he described on tape, groping women without their consent or desire. But the breaking news didn't put me in the corner. The news didn't make me flashback and vomit and sob until I became too dehydrated to produce tears.

It was my Facebook newsfeed that did that.

Because it was there that I saw good, kind, moral individuals who love Jesus defending what Donald Trump described on tape. I saw people I love and respect dismissing concern and outrage over the acts he described. I saw good people decrying those who were upset as being "too sensitive" and overreactive. It was just a few vulgar words, after all.

"It's not the vulgarity," I whisper. "He's describing assault."

And he was. If it happened as he said, he was describing assault. He was describing abuse of power. He was describing victimization that can leave permanent scars. He was describing the sort of event that broke my world and shattered my mind. And in a loud, clear voice, conservative America took to the internet to defend him.

Now it's October 2017 and the internet is ablaze with #MeToo. Thousands upon thousands of people utilize social media to validate the prevalence of sexual assault and harassment. They share their experiences from Hollywood, the boardroom, the schoolroom. And they name names.

I have names I could name. But I don't. I say #MeToo and the messages from fellow survivors, men and women, begin to pour in. Truly, an invisible army of those harmed by sexual assault exists alongside the rest of the world. And if that's the case, how did I find myself in the same position once again, fielding a litany of hurtful, dismissive, skeptical Facebook posts from people who are *kind*? People who would never purposefully hurt someone who is suffering. People who love Jesus and want to walk like him.

I watch as my pastor processes #MeToo and #ChurchToo. He puts out a plea on Facebook. He asks survivors and anyone else with experience dealing with sexual assault and willing to talk to him to please do so. He wants to understand this issue—to make his church a place that's a haven, a place where the Gospel of Jesus Christ is lived out in truth and light.

But does that mean the same church should be a safe place for survivors and perpetrators looking to change? Does a single church congregation have to be both to truly represent the Gospel? Though he listened to my experiences and, I believe, heard my concerns, our conversation triggers me so thoroughly, I'm almost unable to function for the next forty-eight hours.

In the coming weeks, I contemplate ending my life because I'm so weary of the pain. I reach out to my friends and my therapist in moments of crisis, but I have to wonder…will this ever end? Will I ever be able to live my life without feeling like I'm being violated, even when no one is touching me?

Welcome to secondary victimization. Or post-crime victimization. Or double victimization. It's the pain that comes after the pain. The psychological assault that occurs when abuse victims are treated with skepticism, blamed for their abuse, dismissed, brushed aside, or otherwise harmed in conjunction with, but secondary to, the initial abuse.

And it can happen to sexual assault victims when the crimes being discussed were not originally perpetrated against them. In other words, I experienced secondary victimization as a result of the groping allegedly committed by Donald Trump, due to the nature of the ensuing discussion. I experienced it again as I watched people tear down #MeToo survivors with verbal attacks. I experience it every time an assault or harassment scandal hits the news and social media conversations explode. I routinely feel molested by my Facebook newsfeed.

It's a bit mind-blowing to truly wrap one's brain around that, but I've lived it too many times to deny that this psychological phenomenon occurs. The emotions wrenched from my heart, and even the physiological responses of my body, as I listen to the conversation surrounding sexual assault and harassment today mirror what I experienced during my molestation thirty years ago.

It pains me to say what I'm about to say because I love the church. I love the church because Jesus loves the church. My very best friends are part of the church. We are Christ's bride, and I consider myself an eternally grateful member of this body. I love the people of God. But here's the truth of my experience: the church is crueler to abuse victims than the world. The church has been a less safe place to share my experiences with childhood sexual abuse and the ensuing fallout in my life than the world. Sometimes I can find more support from random people on Twitter than I can from my beloved brothers and sisters in Christ when discussing how this abuse still affects me.

Secondary victimization can occur anywhere, but it takes on a particular hue in American Christendom. Well-meaning Christians demand that abuse victims forgive their perpetrators immediately, especially when the perpetrator was a professing Christian. If you don't believe me, observe what happens when a prominent pastor is accused of—or even proven to have com-mitted—sexual misconduct. If the abuse is even brought into the open, the congregation often circles the wagons and protects the pastor, the church, and, they say, the reputation of the church at large. They pronounce the perpetrator healed, demand immediate and complete forgiveness from his victims, and restore him to a position of power. And that's *if* it's brought into the open.

Often, these matters are dealt with quietly. Even when someone stands accused of a crime, authorities are not contacted. Truly independent investigations are rare. Care for the victim falls by the wayside as the church wonders how best to do damage control.

There are probably a hundred different cultural reasons why these particular types of secondary victimization occur in faith communities. We're wary of gossip, and scandals lend themselves well to plenty of gossip. Grace, forgiveness, and mercy are cornerstones of our faith, so perhaps we bend toward immediate forgiveness when that's easiest—when the truth or seeking justice would be painful, difficult, and messy. Which it usually is. Sometimes, I think it's hard for us to believe—maybe even impossible to fathom—the depths of depravity required to sexually victimize someone. Or maybe it's the opposite. Maybe we're keenly aware of our own weaknesses and are terrified of the idea of pulling sin into the light, lest our sin be exposed in the same way.

A frequent refrain I saw from believers during the initial #MeToo explosion in Hollywood was, "Well, of course this is happening in Hollywood. Look how sinful a place it is. They're so liberal there." I wanted to scream. This happens in churches, too. It happens in places where everyone professes to love and follow Jesus. This is not an issue of women placing themselves in an environment that's "sinful anyway" and therefore experiencing violation. These violations occur *everywhere*. Friends, they occurred in my preschool.

Unless we believe sexual violation occurred in that preschool-daycare center back in 1985 because the director was too liberal or the toys in the toy boxes were too racy, at some point we must acknowledge sexual abuse occurs anywhere man's sin nature exists. It happens anywhere power can be abused. And that means it happens everywhere.

I wish I had a neat action plan to share. I wish I had some bullet points. Handling the sexual trauma of others in twelve easy steps, or something like that. I don't. As I told my pastor, I don't really know what the answer is. I don't know how to make victims feel safe while allowing for the possibility of forgiveness and restoration for truly repentant perpetrators.

All I can do is urge my brothers and sisters in Christ to handle sexual assault survivors with care. Listen to our stories. Hear our hearts and understand that a week-long news cycle item for most people is a lifelong component of our stories. Not a day passes that I don't deal in one way or another with my abuse. That's partially because I have chosen to speak about it, hoping to serve as a voice of understanding for others who are struggling. But part of that is because my brain was wired a particular way due to my abuse. I will be working to rewire my thinking and change my patterns for the rest of my life. So when I say "every day," I mean *every single day.*

Trauma survivors are bruised reeds. We are smoldering wicks. Your words have the power to break and snuff. Please use them wisely.

A Little Less Alone

by Stephanie Monk Guido

"I think you need medication."

I still vividly recall the first time my husband spoke those words to me. The room seemed to spin around me; I felt like I'd been verbally slapped. My spine stiffened, and I spit out my reply through clenched teeth.

"How dare you say that to me!"

I turned on my heel and stomped out of the room. Sobbing on my bed, I asked myself what would ever induce a loving person to say such a hateful thing—to question my mental stability?

What I didn't know then was that it was my own preconceptions that made my husband's statement such a hateful thing. My own prejudices that correlated taking an antidepressant with diminished self-worth.

That conversation led to a crying, panicky mother bringing her almost one-year-old to an appointment with a physician's assistant, filling out a post-partum depression questionnaire on the floor of an office meeting room while her baby crawled around and tried to pull things out of the trashcan.

The PA just stared at that distraught mother and tried to keep the baby out of trouble while the mom sobbed out her answers. In her best clinical voice, the PA told the mom that she tested just over the borderline for PPD and handed her a prescription for Zoloft. "Don't worry, PPD is a short-term thing," she said as she ushered the mom out the door.

I hardly recognize myself as that mom. What I can never

forget is the condescension in the PA's voice. The message I took home—a message I hope she didn't intend to give—was that I was temporarily broken, but at least I wasn't broken long-term like some people.

I took the lowest possible dose of the medication, 25mg—like she said, I was only borderline, right? And in three months I was feeling pretty normal. I weaned off and proudly put away the prescription bottle for good. Looking back, I never even took a therapeutic dose, 50mg. A psychiatrist would have known that anything less than a therapeutic dose hadn't really helped; PPD generally disappears on its own. But I never would have been caught dead in a psychiatrist's office back then.

———————

Skip forward one year.

My husband and I had been doing marriage counseling for a couple weeks. Every Friday-morning session dredged up years of old hurts, and our grad-student counselor would wrap up each session with an attempt to tie up the loose strings that were splayed across the ground like a crushed bug.

I'd smile and nod and thank her for her time. If I was lucky, I was able to dog-paddle out of the flood of my emotions by the end of the weekend.

A sunny Saturday morning in February, my world fell apart. My body trembled uncontrollably; I couldn't catch my breath. My heart pounded; a strange terror roared through my body. Every time I thought I'd got it under control, the sight of my two kids and their playmate, the sound of my husband working on his remodeling project, or the memory of that first trembling terror sent me fleeing back into a puddle on the bathroom floor—door locked, air vent on, sobbing like my dad had died.

I managed to dial my friend's number. When she picked up, I gasped for breath. "I think I'm having a panic attack. What do I do?"

Calm and collected, she walked me through some simple steps, asked if I wanted her to come over, and asked if I was okay. I nodded furiously, coughed, and said, "No, I'll be fine. I've got this now."

I didn't. I didn't have it the next time it happened. Or the next. By April, they happened without fail every Thursday night before counseling. Sometimes Wednesday night too. I asked our marriage counselor about it, but it wasn't really in her purview. She recommended a separate counselor.

My husband knew nothing about panic attacks, nor did my family—though I was too embarrassed to admit it to them anyway. I grew more and more petrified, unable to really share what was happening with friends and family. It was too confusing, too embarrassing, and talking about it guaranteed a fresh panic attack.

I made an appointment with a psychiatrist—I was truly desperate by now—and he suggested an antidepressant accompanied by a small bottle of Ativan to take whenever a panic attack struck—but not too often or I'd become dependent. But the Ativan didn't seem to have much impact on my panic attacks. I grew more convinced that nothing and no one could control them.

Then came the Thursday night when I left a favorite group activity early. The panic attack was so strong that I never should have driven myself home. But my mind was so full of terror, I couldn't think clearly to ask someone to help.

My husband and I had been arguing even more lately. I didn't know how to tell him what was going on inside me. With our counseling sessions growing increasingly antagonistic, I couldn't admit there was something terribly wrong with me—that would discount all my emotions past and present, right? Perhaps I really was going crazy.

I barely got the kids to daycare the next morning. I sat outside our counseling session lobby and tried to journal, tried to listen to music, but I just couldn't sit still. My husband arrived, and I raised bloodshot eyes. "I'm not okay. I don't know what to do, but I'm not okay."

———————

This started the week from hell—the week-long panic attack from hell. I later learned I was experiencing rolling panic attacks where the first one doesn't have time to end before the next one begins, then the next one, and the next one. I'd already been struggling to eat, struggling to sit still, waking up early and tired but unable to sleep. At first, I celebrated losing weight. Then, I started forcing myself to at least sip at protein drinks to keep from feeling too sick to move. Because I had to move.

The only times I felt normal were when I was walking outside. Sunday, a week from the start of the panic attack, I walked six miles round-trip. I hadn't eaten anything all day. Or rather, I had, but I'd thrown up breakfast. At the three-mile mark, I stopped and bought a bag of chips. I ate as I walked home. The best food I'd eaten in days.

The next morning was the worst yet. I woke up sobbing. "I

can't do this anymore!" I cried into my husband's shirt. "I just want to die. Why can't I just die?"

We left the kids with friends and headed to the ER. I needed help. Now. And I didn't care how I got it, or how much it cost. No more wait-lines to get in to see doctors, no more slow trials to see what a new medication might do. I had to have relief, if there was any out there. Something I doubted more and more each day.

I jumped at the offer of an inpatient clinic. The woman who would have cowered in terror at the thought of a mental institution only weeks before was now ready to sign any paperwork necessary to get nonstop psychiatric care, new medications at high doses until we found the right one, the promise of solutions. Sign. Me. Up.

Peace. That first night all I felt was the blissful peace of strong benzodiazepines. They checked my blood pressure carefully and had me drink more water to try to bump up my numbers. But nothing could stress me out now. I just floated in the quiet joy of resting, eating, sleeping. I was okay. And, for the first time in months, I truly felt like me.

I think that first night was when it started to hit me. This was the real me. The happy, peaceful, joking girl who jumped for joy when the chocolate came out and stayed up late in bed reading a good book. That panic-ridden, non-stop pacing, suicidal shade of a person? That was a panic disorder running rampant in my system.

Then I started to really look around at the other people in the clinic with me. Since childhood I'd been terrified of mental institutions, picturing them as places where crazy, scary, disturbing people lurked. That was a lie. A big fat lie.

What I saw here in the clinic were some of the bravest people I'd ever met. People who fought the most difficult internal battles I'd ever encountered and had the courage to come get help. Many of them were successful business people, A-grade students, loving moms, and devoted husbands. Their lives looked normal from the outside. But here I was privileged to see the biggest battles they fought—and lost, and won, and fought again.

I started the journey of reconsidering every preconception I held about mental illness. Now that I'd fallen straight into my worst nightmare about mental health, I at last had the courage to look mental illness straight in the face. And the face I saw wasn't a Medusa's head that turned me to stone. Granted, it wasn't a beautiful Madonna face either. But it was a fierce, battle-scarred, fighting face—an admirable and awesome sight.

And now I was part of the fighting team, and proud of it. Dealing with mental health issues is no fun. Remember my story? It was hell. And that story continues, and it can still be hellish. But it's no longer something that makes me ashamed.

When I left the clinic four days later, I felt stronger than I ever had before—but also more fragile. I started putting my mental health needs first, and that meant saying "no" when I used to say "yes." It meant waiting in the car if I felt overwhelmed at a social function or hiding in the bathroom if necessary. It meant deciding to go exercise or spend an evening reading in my room if I couldn't handle my children's high energy at the moment.

Those choices were easy. The hard part was combating the lies my brain told me, lies that many of us know all too well. And they have nothing to do with my panic disorder. They're lies that say: you're selfish, you're not a good friend, and you're not a good mother.

That last one was the hardest for me. How could I be a good mother when I couldn't always be there for my kids? What kind of mother sometimes didn't have anything left to give her kids emotionally? What kind of mother stepped away when her kids were needy and took care of herself first?

A wise mother. Not the mother of society's idealization, but a mother who knows herself and her boundaries well enough to make the best choice.

And in rushed the stream of society's expectations. Fresh from my journey toward changing my own prejudices, I ran smack dab into the middle of society's prejudices.

I grew up in church. I'd heard all the lies—depression is always a spiritual issue, good Christians don't have mental health problems, you don't need medication, just prayer.

But I also grew up in a wise, loving, Christian family, and they spoke truth; they rejected these lies. They had been nothing but supportive from the moment they found out what I was dealing with. My family prayed, they encouraged, they rejoiced with me when a new medication worked. They researched medication side effects and helped me make choices. They went to doctor appointments with me. They were a godsend.

As I walked back into my life with a purse full of new prescriptions, I found myself faced with a choice I'd completely lost sight of in the haze of sickness. What was I going to tell my friends? Acquaintances? Strangers? It's not like you can simply slip away because of a panic attack and nobody will notice. When you're having a panic attack in the middle of a shopping trip, what do you tell the cashier when you can't seem to get your credit card out of your wallet?

This launched me into another brand-new world—being an amateur mental health education specialist. I started telling people exactly what was happening to me when my panic attacks came. This involved a lot of explanation and research. Now I can answer questions about panic disorders, anxiety disorders, panic attacks, psychiatrists, psychologists, psychiatric medication, and side effects.

I've talked to numerous students and parents in high school courses I've taught, and I've been thrilled to be able to share my story as they struggle to navigate the path of mental health issues. What breaks my heart, though, is how often I hear that I'm the only person they've talked to who really seems to understand and who identifies with how isolating mental health issues are. The only one who knows how scary it is to talk about and how unsafe it feels to admit anything's wrong. The only one who's lived through it and rejects the stigma.

I consider it my sacred privilege to educate people about mental health issues, to do my part to take away the stigma. Every time a person's eyes widen as they realize this perfectly normal twenty-something mother deals with mental health issues, I pray they take a step closer to realizing that my struggle doesn't make me strange or untrustworthy. It doesn't make me weird.

The greatest honor, though, has been to talk to fellow fighters. My chest warms with empathy when I explain to a new friend that I'm feeling panicky because I forgot to take my medication, and she looks at me with wonder and admits that she takes an antidepressant too. We jump into talking shop about medications and side effects, and I find that, in a struggle that stigmatizes its sufferers, one more person feels a little less alone.

I Thought I Was Normal

by Joel Larson

I believed I was normal and among the seventy-five percent of people who do not struggle with mental illness. After all, I was a chaplain assistant. I was in the military. I was a pastor. I have an advanced degree in the Bible. I was a crisis counselor. I am the spiritual director for a mental health hospital system. I don't fit the profile. But my history says otherwise.

My story started in 2005 with a deployment to Iraq as an Army chaplain assistant. On March 31, 2005, I was standing on the front steps of my chapel when a mortar round came in and blew up a generator across the street. I don't think I have ever been that scared in my life, but I did my job and helped care for the wounded.

A few weeks later, I was on a patrol with a group of Iraqi police trainees when shots were fired near us. I can honestly say that it took years to remember everything that happened that day because I went into autopilot.

And then I flew home for my Rest and Recuperation (R&R). It was a wonderful time for my family. My second son was born while I was home and we celebrated. Then the R&R was over, and I started my flight back to Iraq. This is where the real adventure began.

A close friend dropped me off at the Phoenix airport and I checked into my flight. As I sat down to wait for my flight, it began to happen. My chest tightened, my legs started to hurt, I started sweating, the world started spinning. I didn't know what was happening.

I loosened my bootlaces, but that didn't help. Now I had to get on the plane and I was still a physical mess. My seat was in the back, by the window, next to a man who used half of my seat—I am not a small guy, so this intensified my discomfort. Needless to say, I couldn't get off that plane fast enough.

Next were a couple hours of waiting in the Dallas-Fort Worth Airport, only I couldn't sit still. I walked the whole time. I ran outside to feel the sunlight, but it was July so the air outside only felt heavy and oppressive. Finally, we got on the plane—it felt like days, not hours. I was lucky, I got an aisle seat, but that didn't help the sweating, the dizziness, the chest pain, or anything else.

The tightness in my chest was unbearable. I couldn't keep my legs still. My world was still spinning. I couldn't sleep all night, so I attempted to walk around the plane. We finally landed in Romania, but we were not allowed to get off the plane. I thought I was going crazy. I wanted to run screaming off the plane, but I couldn't—they wouldn't let us.

I think at this point that I had been awake for about twenty-four hours, but I was too tired to sleep and I still couldn't sit still. My legs ached and my chest was still tight. We finally got back in the air and landed in Kuwait. I felt some relief because we are able to get off the plane and walk around, but only for a moment. Everyone piled in a bus, filled every seat, bags on our laps. The feelings came back—tightness, dizziness, achiness, panic. I continued to ask myself, "Am I crazy? What is this feeling?"

I hooked up with some members of my unit who left Phoenix the day before and we caught an early flight back to Iraq—maybe not the best choice in retrospect. I got back on a plane, my fourth flight, and everything came back. My brain hurt, my legs were restless, and my chest felt tight. I wondered, "Am I dying?" I had been up for about thirty-six hours.

We finally landed in Iraq. After getting my weapon, I walked back to my Containerized Housing Unit (CHU). I wanted to take a quick shower and maybe catch a short nap before getting back to work (I think I had been up about forty-eight hours by now). However, I couldn't sit still or close my eyes. My chest was tight, the world was spinning, and my CHU was collapsing on me. I got dressed and went to my chapel to check in.

They asked, "What are you doing here? Go get some rest."

"I can't rest, I am pacing and I feel like I am going crazy. Why won't the thoughts stop? What is wrong with me?"

The chaplain I worked with took me to the hospital. "You might be dehydrated. Drink some water and see what happens. You will be fine."

After dinner, things began to normalize for me, but the tightness in my chest was still there, reminding me that I wasn't okay yet. I tried to stay outside. It felt so good outside. The world stopped spinning. For a moment anyway.

I had a staff meeting that I needed to attend. I went, and the room felt like it was falling in on me. I couldn't handle it anymore. Finally, the meeting was done, and I was able to go to my CHU. It was time to get a good night's sleep. I think I had been up about fifty-four hours by then.

However, I still couldn't sleep. Everything ramped up again—dizziness, chest tightness, the CHU falling inward on me, terror. I wanted to run and scream, but where would I go? There was nowhere.

I went back to the emergency room, because it was the only

place I felt safe all day. They gave me an anti-anxiety medication and told me to get some sleep. By the time I finally fell asleep, I had been awake for fifty-six hours—most of that time in a full panic attack.

I got referred to the psychiatrist. "What happened?" he asked. "Where do you think it came from?"

I felt like an idiot. I was supposed to be strong. I was supposed to be able to handle stress. I couldn't even sit in an office without having a panic attack. I was diagnosed with anxiety disorder unspecified.

"Have you ever felt like this before?"

The easy answer was yes. The hard part was identifying when it began. I started to analyze my life. I thought back through college, the Army, basic training, high school, middle school, elementary school, Fort Huachuca, Fort Devens, and Germany. Then it hit me—the first time I felt this way.

I was five years old and needed to have some dental work done. I don't even remember what they were doing, but because it was painful, the dentist strapped me into a papoose board. I couldn't move. And I felt my chest tighten and my legs began to hurt and I wanted to run away screaming.

The psychiatrist gave me prescriptions for Xanax and Ativan. "Just take the drugs and things will be better."

I am not sure if you know what Xanax does to you, but it is not a feeling you want when you're in a combat situation. I couldn't bring myself to take it.

My chaplain, my spiritual advisor at the time, was not much help either. "It is a psychological problem. Listen to the psychiatrist. He knows what to do. I don't have any idea how to help you. You just need to be ready if something happens."

———————

When I got back to the States, everything felt wrong. I left with one child, I came home to two. My wife sold our home while I was gone, and we were renting the house we once owned while a new house was being built. I didn't fit in at work, my marriage felt like a wreck, my oldest son barely recognized me and certainly didn't know me.

Everything felt wrong.

I was a hero at my church; I gave up parts of my life so that others could experience freedom. Only I didn't feel like a hero. No, I felt like my life was falling apart.

I went back to work in 2006, but something was different. I can look back now and tell you that I was experiencing depression, but then, I did not know what it was. All I knew was this: I was struggling with reintegrating with my family, I was experiencing triggers from my time in Iraq, and I was angry at everything.

In 2008, my wife and I felt God tell us that the church we were helping to lead needed to close and He was going to move us in a new direction. Of course, I knew what that direction was, and so I started heading that way. I just *knew* that God wanted me to be an administrative pastor for a church; unfortunately, I was wrong.

I was always the guy who just applied for a job and got it. There was never any real competition. So when I received my first rejection letter, I was devastated. Looking back, I felt like God rejected me. My second rejection letter was even worse. Nevertheless, I started seminary during this same season.

I don't know what I thought seminary would be like, but it

was hard work. I started in January 2009, going to school full time, working full time, and…being a not-very-good father and husband. I was still very angry at everything. I continued to apply for pastoral positions but continued to get rejected.

In October 2010, three years of nonstop stress began. I can't say that I ever felt better, or that I recovered in any way from my depression, but I kept plugging along because I believed that God was taking me somewhere and I knew that it was going to be a great place.

The first thing that happened was that my mother went into congestive heart failure. She was in the ICU in Tucson for over a month. During that time, I commuted from Phoenix to Tucson about two or three times a week, completed a Greek class, completed an Old Testament class, continued working full time, and helped to lead a small group at my church. I know that my work suffered and I am pretty sure that everything else did, too. I have to say that I wondered what God would throw at me next.

A few months later, we found out that our dog had lymphoma. It was bad, and I had to take him to the vet and have him put to sleep. This was the first time I had ever done anything like that. It was the worst day of my life up to that point. Eight months later, we put our second dog to sleep for a different type of cancer. The process of putting down our second dog might have been easier or it might have been harder, but I still don't know if I can tell you. My heart still aches when I think about my puppies.

What I remember most now is that I had lost my faith and trust in humanity. And maybe, I lost faith in God too.

In May 2011, I hit rock bottom professionally. The church that I was managing hosted a conference with many moving parts and I ended up managing many of those moving parts. They wanted daily newsletters, signs, and advertisements, plus we needed to keep the church running because we were still going to have church on Sunday. The stress got to be too much and I snapped. The anger got the best of me and I realized something—I did not know who I was anymore. Something had to change.

Thankfully, that change was on the way. Only a few weeks later, the Senior Chaplain for the Arizona National Guard called me and wanted to know if I would take an active duty tour. They were rolling out a new program for increasing resilience in soldiers and they had lots of money to spend. I thought this might be my chance to get out of a work situation I did not want to be in and make a new start, so I agreed. I thought this might fix all my problems.

Shortly after I accepted the role, I learned about a new program called Combat and Operational Stress First Aid, for which the Arizona National Guard needed instructors. I was able to get trained and began learning about the effects of stress on the human body. However, I did not notice or understand my own stressors. I did not know it then, but this would become a very important teaching and program in my life.

Things went well for a while in our family. We were able to find a new church, finances seemed to take care of themselves, my wife and I began to get along better, and my kids started in Cub Scouts. Life seemed normal. Until the wheels fell off again.

In March 2012, once again, I had the wind knocked out of my sails. My mother called me and informed me that in order to live, she would need to get a heart transplant and she would need to fight to get it. I know now I was pretty angry with God for this at the time, but I am pretty sure I didn't realize it in the moment.

Over the course of the next five months, my mother would

be in and out of hospitals in Sierra Vista, Tucson, and Phoenix. She would end up at the Mayo Hospital in North Phoenix. I was continuing to teach about Stress First Aid, work for the National Guard, attend seminary, lead Cub Scouts, be a father, and be a husband. All the while ignoring the warning signs of anxiety and depression in my own life.

————————

It was July 24, 2012, and I got a call from my father that I needed to come to the hospital. My mother was not doing well. My kids were at a National Guard kids' Lego event. I had to pull them out. I headed north to the Mayo Hospital and found out what was wrong.

She had a massive heart attack and they had to do CPR to bring her back. She was stable but not doing well. We called for my brother to come home from Texas where he was stationed with the Army. Mayo would not let us stay overnight, so we went home.

We drove back first thing in the morning with all the kids. We hoped that if she saw her grandkids, it would give her even more reason to fight. But Mayo would not let the kids go in and see her; she was too compromised for them to visit. My brother and his wife visited her first. My sister and her husband went in second. My father visited her third. My wife and I were last.

She signed "I love Jesus." While we were there, a look of pain came across her face and she grabbed her chest. The monitors went crazy; the nurses rushed in; my wife pulled me out and I stood in the hallway. My wife told me that we needed to leave, so we walked out to the waiting room. I followed numbly, not quite sure what was happening but fearing the worst.

The adults decided it was time for the kids to go home. I didn't know what to do, so I went down to the chapel and cried out to God in a way I had never cried out before. It didn't work. She passed after a massive heart attack.

My mother passed on a Thursday morning and three days later, I was in church. I was watching my kids singing in their vacation Bible school celebration and all of a sudden, it hit me: "My mother will never see this again." I lost it. I couldn't control my emotions, I ran out of the church sobbing. One of my friends came out, placed his hand on my shoulder and told me, "God always has a purpose for these things." It didn't help.

I dealt with the funeral and began to move forward with my life, but nothing seemed to have purpose. What were we working for anyway? Two months later, September 25, a family friend passed away. I felt nothing but darkness around me, but I kept moving blindly forward. Finally, my cat was killed. I would like to say that this was the final straw, but there was still more to come.

I was in my last year of seminary and completing an internship that required a weekly meeting with a mentor. I chose a pastor friend who should have helped me move toward my calling to pastor. He didn't; instead, we ended up talking every week about how terrible his church plant was going and how much he hated Phoenix.

But the hits kept coming. I was taking a class on pastoral ministries. This class was intended to teach us how to be better pastors and care for people. One night, our professor was talking about counseling people, and he stated he believed depression is a sin.

I could not believe it. I was suffering in a dark place, I didn't know what God was doing, and this man told me that depression is a sin. What he really told me that night was far worse—that I was not good enough to be a pastor because I was struggling with sin. But I couldn't control this supposed sin. I could control other sins, but not this one. I wanted to run screaming from class or give this professor a piece of my mind, but instead I did nothing. Why bother?

Finally, in the middle of November 2012, I was told that the Arizona National Guard was running out of money for the resilience program and I was going to lose my job. My last day on orders was December 31, 2012.

So, in the previous two years, I had lost three animals, my mother, and a job. I was in a pretty bad spot. So I did what I needed to do. I began working on my resume and started applying for jobs. One rejection after another came in, and I started wondering what I was going to do. Was I not good enough to do anything? No one wanted me as a pastor, no one wanted me as a manager, and no one wanted me as a salesman. What exactly was left that I was qualified for?

After a particularly bad job interview, I was driving home. I looked at an overpass and the concrete columns holding up the bridge and thought, "I have over a million dollars in life insurance. My family would totally be taken care of if I died." And I scared the crap out of myself.

I think that was one of the longest nights of my life. I talked with my wife and a close friend about the thoughts I was having. I was crying out and the only people who could help me were my wife, my friend, and my psychologist. This time, she sent me to my primary care physician to put me on antidepressants.

At this point in the story, I need to go back a step and talk about my mentoring relationship. As we were meeting each week, I would talk about how useless and worthless life felt. My mentor's responses communicated to me that these feelings were wrong and not Christian. He told me, "Don't let them put you on those drugs. They are bad and will turn you into a zombie."

The next week, I was feeling suicidal and the doctors were telling me I needed to take medications. Who should I believe? Who had my best interests in mind? I decided I needed to take the medication.

The day of my next appointment with my psychologist, I talked with a friend who worked for a company that provided on-site mobile crisis counseling. She asked if I had a job yet. When I said no, she picked up her cell phone and started to make a call.

She finished the phone call and said, "I have a job for you. Send your resume to this email address."

When I told her I was not prepared for that, she told me not to worry. I received a call about two hours later asking me if I would come in for a job interview the next day.

The following morning, I had my appointment with my primary care physician and was prescribed antidepressants, then went directly to the job interview. Before the interview was over, they were asking me about Combat and Operational Stress First Aid and how to incorporate that training into their crisis response teams. They almost offered me a job on the spot, but they needed to check my references. I started that job about three weeks later.

In December 2012, I started working as a mobile crisis counselor going out into people's homes, public spaces, restaurants, and even gas stations to help people who were struggling with mental health issues, suicidal thoughts, and homicidal thoughts.

In June 2013, I graduated from seminary and earned a Masters of Divinity degree. I was promoted to a crisis therapist position, and I was responsible for a crisis team helping people in the community. What a far cry from the office manager role I held a few short years before.

About six months later, I received a phone call from the senior chaplain at a local hospital. He told me that a behavioral health system of hospitals wanted to create a chaplain program and I needed to send them my resume. And that's where I am today. I am the spiritual director for a mental health hospital system. I invest each day in providing a safe space for those fighting the same battles I still face myself.

As a chaplain, I talk to people who have been told that they are demon possessed and need an exorcism. I find their demons are the abuse they have suffered or the trauma they have experienced that their brain reminds them of at the most inopportune times.

I have talked with people who have told me that their pastor told them that they should not take psychiatric medications, because they block the power of the Holy Spirit. Instead, if they just had enough faith in God, they would be healed. As Christians, we need to do better at understanding mental health and caring for those in our midst who are struggling. Mental illness is not a sin. And medication for mental illness can be effective. Christians, especially pastors, need to be informed and trained about mental illness. We need to love "the least of these…" And that includes those who are dealing with mental illness.

And do you know what I think scares me the most about this story? I realized as I wrote it that I am the one in four. I struggle with a mental illness. I struggle with depression. Sometimes, I do not want to get up in the morning, and sometimes I feel the dark cloud following me, and sometimes I do not want to deal with other people. I am still in the midst of the battle.

But we can make a difference, and by sharing our stories, we can help the church understand. One story at a time.

SCARED OF MY OWN VOICE

BY JANEEN IPPOLITO

For so long, no one spoke up for me.

Not enough. Not in ways that mattered.

Speaking is held in such high regard in the church. We are called to watch our words wisely and be careful what we say. Never lie, never condemn. Let God be the judge.

But I never heard a single sermon about fathers screaming at their children or treating them unjustly—and I've been to a lot of services across many denominations. No, in every sermon I heard words about overlooking offenses. About giving unreasonable grace and mercy, just like Christ did.

Some of the pastors screamed as loud as he did. I assumed it was normal for some men. Acceptable. It showed their passion, their focus. Some men, the pulpit implied, were simply so powerful that they couldn't contain their zeal. And they shouldn't have to.

The hour-long and two-hour-long tirades showed he cared. Somehow. I just couldn't see it.

No one told me something was wrong with him until I was a teenager. Even then, no conclusive words were used, only hinted at. OCD. Anxiety. Possibly bipolar. By then, the damage had been done.

It didn't matter what anyone told me. In my heart, I knew that my role was to listen quietly, no matter how much anger or hurt or violence came from his mouth. I knew not to tell anyone.

It was the worst-kept family secret, but somehow, it would only reflect badly on us if I said something.

The homes of my relatives and friends were safe. I hoped no one noticed that I cringed every time someone raised their voice. That I was scared of my own voice.

My own shouting was an inexcusable curse, a sign that I would be just like him and hurt others.

Sticks and stones hurt, but words?

They shatter you from the inside out in places you feel weak to admit to. So you don't admit to the pain. You get stronger. You build up wall after wall after wall. Brick by brick, mortared with the resolve that in enduring the abuse of others, you are somehow holier.

It didn't help that the moods changed. That sometimes, especially in public, he was friendly and disarmingly awkward. That some days he reached for the sky with wild excitement and adventure. That he would give anyone the shirt off his back and far more. That he would give you his time and listen to every care and concern you had.

Sometimes, he was the most loving man I had ever met.

But every gift came with a price. A thick, invisible chain that meant I was his. In order to enjoy his highs, I had to suffer his lows and endure every screaming fit. If I fled, retribution would be waiting for me, as would his threats to reveal every single secret I had told him, secrets he held tight and used to control me whenever he decided the punishment was fair and just.

Then, at the darkest moment when I could take no more, the madhouse would spin a different direction. Up was down and down was up, and suddenly he was the victim and I the unfair, sinful, evil accuser. The ungracious. The unforgiving.

Every single buzzword I heard from the pulpit.

And so, I gave in to the emotional abuse. No one had told me to do otherwise. During my childhood I had been offered safe spaces and comfort. Weekend respites and veiled looks of understanding.

But no one ever dared to counter the lies he spoke with truth. I learned how I should pity his mental infirmities and pray for his daily struggles and strive not to take it personally. That I should open my arms to the thorn-like words, buried deep into my skin and blood and heart. It was my Christian duty to endure underneath the pain of assault.

After all, he had never laid a hand on me. He had only prevented me from leaving a room. Threatened harm to himself if I turned away.

The absence of physical strikes meant I hadn't been abused.

So I built my walls higher and tighter. I held back more and more trust, not only from him but from the world around me, even from my closest friends. I spread the lies I was taught to others. The lie that coping with the verbal onslaught somehow sanctified me. The lie that because of his mental illness he could never be held culpable. Mercy would never allow me to speak to legal professionals or counselors. That could damage him even further.

They say actions speak louder than words. In this case, it was the inaction and the enabling words of my church brothers and sisters that told me my wounds meant nothing because I wasn't mentally ill. I believed those actions and words with my whole heart, and in turn, believed it was God's will that I continue to face abuse.

I only waited for the day when God Himself would smite me, as fathers did.

Until the day I finally broke. Until the day someone close to me caught me hiding in a closet with my phone, tears streaming down my face as I bravely endured another round of verbal ferocity from my father's bad day.

That family member fought for me. Pushed aside the lies that came from my mouth, the insistence that I was fine. That this is what children endured for their fathers. Children stayed present for their fathers, no matter the abuse and life-altering trauma that resulted.

With gentle words as firm as iron, they tore down every excuse and spoke truth. They never blamed me or thought for a moment that I somehow deserved or asked for the abuse. They were patient with each brainwashed phrase that emerged from my mouth and counteracted each one with the love of Christ.

They stood in the gap and got involved, even when it meant facing that abuse themselves. They advocated for me in our church, a church with a counselor on staff to intervene and guide. One who told me that nothing in Scripture endorsed my father's actions. One who believed verbal abuse was real.

It was the first time I realized a church cared about words, not merely actions.

Since then, time and distance and many caring people have helped me heal. I have learned respect for myself and when to turn away from abuse. I have learned that I have my own neurological differences that make processing difficult situations even harder. I have learned to stand in the strength gained from years of conflict and trauma. I have learned the firm, gentle words to turn away the wrath of others.

I have gained confidence in my voice. I have become a leader, a promoter of good and true words. A believer in others when they can't believe in themselves.

And yet.

Confrontations still make me shake deep into the night when only my spouse can see. I still breathe a sigh of relief after I challenge someone, and they don't prevent me from leaving the room. Occasionally, I still have nightmares. The worst sort, mixed with my father's incredible kindness and the intense attacks and abuse.

I still sit in church every Sunday, hearing sermons preached against physical abuse but never against verbal or emotional abuse. Sermons where congregants are encouraged to care for the mentally ill but never to hold them accountable for their actions. It seems the mentally ill are either saintly angels or abominable demons. Never sinners like the rest of us who have their own inclinations toward good and evil. Never people who can show untold kindness to strangers and rip their own offspring to shreds.

The mentally ill have many struggles. But while having compassion for those struggles, the church cannot overlook or dismiss the damage some mentally ill people can have on others. In attempting to protect one, they cannot allow the harm of another.

An imbalance in the brain is a poor bandage to the scars of verbal and emotional abuse.

I implore church officials to listen to all sides of the story. To indeed, care for the mentally ill and have grace for them as they would for all who struggle.

And yet.

Remember that mental illness does not have to go hand in hand with abuse—but it can. Remember to speak out against verbal and emotional abuse as strongly as physical abuse.

To speak.

You never know who is listening, how your words could touch their hearts and cause them to act. To believe in themselves.

To know there is a safe place.

To know they are not alone.

SOMETHING THAT WILL NOT LET GO

BY ANONYMOUS

He picked me out of a roomful of Sunday school children.

I was only eight years old, and I've sometimes wondered why he chose me. Did he believe I would be easy to control, or that I wouldn't tell anyone? Perhaps he sensed an opportunity, as he was friends with my family. Regardless, the first time he raped me was in my bedroom in the middle of the night, mere yards down the hall from where my parents were sleeping. After that, he became my babysitter and continued to rape me. He said that if I told my parents, they would be angry with me and blame me. I was confused and scared. I didn't understand what he was doing to me. Something told me it was wrong, but I didn't know if I was to blame or not. I kept my silence until, at nine years old, I told the pastor's son what had happened.

I thought it was the right thing to do, but one of the older children in the church who overheard me told me that I shouldn't have said anything. He said it in such a way that I was afraid for what might happen to me, afraid that the rapist had told me the truth: I had done something wrong and now I was going to get in trouble. I wanted to take back my words, but it was too late. A dreadful fear filled me as I stood in the back of the church and watched the pastor's son tell his parents what I'd said.

As it turned out, the rapist was right.

What followed next would forever change the course of my life. It would change the very nature of my being. My family and church would become one intertwined unit and make choices that haunt me to this day.

My mother took me aside when no one else was in the house. She put me on her lap, facing me away from her, and asked me a couple of brief questions about what had happened. At that time, I didn't know she already knew—that she had found the bloody sheets from the first time I had been raped. I was terrified. Everything the rapist had said was coming true. She was cold and distant toward me. I wasn't allowed to look at her. Though she didn't blame me in words, her demeanor convinced me that what the rapist had done to me was my fault. I was so afraid of what she was going to do, that in telling her what had happened, I also told her that he hit me. I knew it was wrong to hit someone, so maybe if she knew he had hit me, she wouldn't be so angry with me.

She said nothing and gave no indication that she cared, and I knew then that I had done something unforgivable, because mothers care. Everyone knows that. But mine didn't. In the course of that short conversation, she never asked me if I was okay or how I was feeling. She never asked me if I had questions. I had so many. She never told me it wasn't my fault. She never told me she loved me. She never hugged me. She never showed any concern at all for what had happened to me. All she did was order me never to tell my father, because he would kill the rapist and go to jail. She then put me down and walked away from me and never brought up the subject again.

I was confused beyond imagining. I didn't understand what the blood meant. I didn't understand what had happened to me. I didn't understand why my father would kill this man when I was the one at fault. As I stood and watched my mother walk away from me, I felt something die inside of me, and I knew I was alone. I would have to take care of myself. The part of me that thought the rapist had done something wrong lay buried under a landslide of guilt and shame, leaving me with a sense of gratitude that I hadn't been punished more harshly than I was.

It was also clear to me that the church didn't care, either. I had told the pastor's son about the rapist and watched him tell his parents, all for nothing. The rapist stayed in the church, where I had to go and see him sitting there. I had to worship with him. I felt him watching me. I was alone and very afraid, and there was nothing else I could do. I knew if I ever spoke of what the rapist did to me again, my father would end up in jail and our family would be destroyed.

That, too, would be my fault.

So in my fear, I smiled and pretended that everything was perfectly fine. When I ate dinner at the rapist's house and sat across the table from him, I smiled and pretended to be happy. When my mother and the pastor's wife talked about the rapist in front of me, something that hurt me deeply, I smiled and pretended all was well. I never once cried, and anytime that I came close to tears, I would scream cruel things at myself inside my head until the feeling went away. Any feeling that might have given me away, I suppressed with an iron will, and I spent the rest of my childhood trying to be good enough to make up for what I had done.

Years later, I learned that others in the church knew I had been raped. They ignored it. Though not well-liked, the rapist came from a prominent family. My mother, the pastor and his wife, and one of the other leaders of the church and his wife decided that reporting the rapist to the authorities would cause too many problems in and for the church, even possibly destroying the church. They swept it neatly under the rug and it became as though it never happened.

Apart from the rapes, my childhood was fairly ordinary, but the rapes overshadowed and permeated everything about me. They haunted me, trailing me like ghosts only I could see. Coping with them was hard enough; the enforced silence oppressed and choked me. Pretending I had not been raped did not make it so. *I* knew what had happened, and I knew *they* knew what had happened. Their silence, lack of compassion, and failure to act told me one thing: it didn't matter. An eight-year-old girl being repeatedly raped by a man in the church did not matter. It wasn't important and it didn't matter and therefore, by extension, I wasn't important. I didn't matter. And, in fact, that was the truth. I *didn't* matter, something I came to believe with all my heart. When something matters, it changes how you act. As the epistle of James makes clear, belief cannot be divorced from action. The church cannot preach that children should be treasured and protected and then choose not to protect them. By choosing not to protect me, they demonstrated what they believed.

Their abandonment forced me to deal with the effects of repeated rape alone. It didn't take long before I developed symptoms of PTSD and showed classic signs of sexual abuse. I became anxious and withdrawn. I had intense feelings of guilt and shame. I had flashbacks and nightmares. I experienced a sudden onset of bedwetting, which prompted my pediatrician to ask me if someone had touched me inappropriately. Terrified, I told him no. And there was a period of inexplicable weight gain. Some of these symptoms I was punished for experiencing. Other symptoms appeared in my young adult years. Many remain with me even now to varying degrees:

- Anxiety and fear
- Guilt and shame
- Hypervigilance
- Difficulty trusting
- Irritability and anger
- Intrusive thoughts
- Nightmares and flashbacks
- Deep-seated feelings of worthlessness

Some symptoms, such as the nightmares and flashbacks, are sporadic; others are more constant. In my nightmares, my family and church together celebrate the rapist and throw parties for him, or they throw parties for me with the rapist as the surprise guest of honor. I walk among them screaming that he is evil and not to be trusted. But I am invisible to everyone but the rapist, and they can't hear me.

There are aspects of the abuse that I can't talk about, or even dwell on in my mind, without inciting a panic attack. Though I have grown into a woman, there is a place deep inside me where, as my counselor put it, dwells the little girl I once was. She lives in a continual state of fear and alertness, as though trapped in a never-ending emergency, and I don't know how to convince her that the danger is over and she is okay. There are certain situations that provoke a fight-or-flight response in me, and other, deeper symptoms that make it likely I will never marry.

Because I had spent so many years suppressing my feelings, I was in my thirties before I understood my need for counseling and talking about what had happened. I was forty when I grieved for the first time what had been done to me and what had been taken from me, when I was finally comfortable acknowledging to myself how worthless I felt. Although I know in my head I did nothing wrong, the guilt and shame linger. The insidious lies I was taught as a child had become my truth for so long, fighting to reclaim myself from those feelings and dismantle those lies has been an uphill and painful battle.

Even as I write this essay, part of me minimizes the trauma. Was it really that bad? I recently read a ten-part journalistic investigation into the sex trafficking of children in the United States and around the world. As I learned about the horrors these precious ones suffer at the hands of the adults in their lives, self-condemnation rose in me. I wasn't sold into the sex trade and raped five times a day like these children are. Am I justified in being upset about what happened? Does it really matter?

Do I really matter?

We're odd creatures, humans. We like to put people and their experiences into boxes. We like to categorize them and label them and assign to each person or experience a measure of our sympathy or judgment in proportion to the box we've put them in. But one person's suffering does not invalidate someone else's. What happened to me matters. I matter, even when I doubt that is true.

And I matter to God—I believe; help my unbelief. I couldn't always see it, especially in the moment, but He cared for me when my family and church did not. I came to faith in Christ prior to having been raped, and His grace carried me through my childhood and sustained me in so many ways. When I was twelve, He sent into my life a girl who became my best friend from the moment we met. She was the only person in my life at that time whom I felt loved me for me. We instantly clicked.

She accepted me for who I was, and I don't think I would have survived adolescence without her.

I found His grace in music that validated my feelings and experiences, such as Plumb and LaRue and Amy Grant and October Project, from whose song "Bury My Lovely" I took the title of this essay. There were TV shows in which evil was punished and children were treasured that gave me strength and hope and helped me connect with people who cared, fictitious though they were. How often I wished that Robert McCall would rescue me, or that I could live in the tunnels beneath New York City with Vincent and Father. And I always had books. In the movie *Shadowlands*, one of C. S. Lewis's students comments, "We read to know we're not alone." This was true for me. For so much of my childhood, I shut myself up in my room, reading. Reading helped me cope. It helped me survive. It provided an escape and connected me to others who understood me. It made me feel less alone. Even today, I find God's grace in song and screen and story.

God also showered me with grace by the people He brought into my life as an adult—wonderful women who mentored me, and sometimes mothered me, who weren't afraid to enter into my messy story, who encouraged me, who supported me, who loved me, who spoke truth to my doubts and comfort to my fears, who painted my story on canvas and sent me gift cards to Applebee's so I could enjoy french fries after a difficult counseling session, who became dear friends I hold in my heart. They are more precious to me than all the world.

But in spite of all this grace, I struggle to believe God loves me and cares about me. I find I can't connect with Him on an emotional level. I can't relate to the verses that speak of His love. I feel like He is often angry and disappointed with me, or has better things than me to concern Himself with. Prayer is difficult and not always my first response to life.

As a child, I would sit in church and study the stained glass that surrounded me. One window depicted the scene from St. Mark's gospel where Jesus takes the children in His arms and blesses them. I tried to imagine what it would be like to be the child cuddled in His arms on His lap, nestled safe against Him. I couldn't. I have no idea what that feels like. Trying to imagine it felt blasphemous, because He would never do that. Not with me.

There are deep, spiritual consequences to abuse.

So what relationship does the church have with trauma survivors who have PTSD? This is not an easy question to answer, because local churches and parishes vary and every survivor's experience will vary. My own experience varies. I know there are wonderful churches that are vigilant protectors of children and safe havens for those with PTSD, but this has generally not been my experience.

The church of my youth suffered from massive failures in leadership. In my early teens, the pastor was sexually inappropriate with me, kissing me as I had seen him kiss his wife. When I finally was able to start processing my past and talk about it, he phoned me, angry and defensive, claiming he never knew that anything had happened to me. Apparently what he did didn't count. At the same time, the other leader and his wife acknowledged knowing that I had been raped. For so many years, I had felt discarded and rejected and abandoned. So intense was my gratitude that someone in the church finally admitted the truth that it was nearly a *decade* before I realized he never offered an apology for his or the church's lack of action at the time. In fact, no one has ever apologized to me for what happened or accepted responsibility for their actions.

I've long since moved away from where I grew up, but occasionally return to visit my sister. I don't know that the church has improved much in that time, even though the leadership has changed. On my last visit, the church was preparing for vacation Bible school. In the most ironic moment I have ever observed, the pastor, standing beneath the image of Jesus holding the children in His arms, warned the congregation to be wary of the children who would attend VBS. They were liars and would claim to be sexually assaulted as a means of extorting money from the church. I was so horrified, I was speechless. I felt nine years old again.

Any healing I have achieved is in spite of this church, not because of it.

I have also had encounters in the church with people who downplay, deny, or criticize mental illness. Sadly, it's a byword in the church that we shoot our wounded. This should not be so. Our wounded should be cherished and cared for. I have also had people in the church, including a counselor, express to me their surprise that the trauma I experienced would still affect me "after all these years." They don't understand PTSD. To mitigate long-term consequences of trauma, it is important to receive treatment as soon as possible. As time passes, memories of the trauma become permanent and impervious to treatment.[1] I received no treatment at all until I sought it out twenty-five years later. Of course it still affects me. There's a chance it always will.

Thankfully, my interactions haven't been wholly negative. My current church is nothing like my former church. It's hard for me to talk about the rapes, but from the tentative feelers I have ex-

---

1   https://www.ncbi.nlm.nih.gov/pmc/articles/PMC3181836/

tended, I have been received with welcome and compassion. My denomination has a ministry dedicated to victims of child abuse. I also have the privilege of being part of an online prayer group that is full of compassion and kindness to the hurting and weary. They have helped me find grace in the mundane, and allowed me to be part of their own messy stories, which is how the church was meant to be.

I have survived, even though some days it doesn't feel like it. My resources for treatment have been limited at times, but I fight for healing, moving forward a tiny step at a time. Though I struggle with many things, I don't desire vengeance. I don't hope or pray that God would harm those who destroyed the life I might have had. Is this forgiveness? I don't know. I've spent my life trying to understand what forgiveness is and how it plays out in practical, real living, but I remain uncertain. It doesn't help that theologians can't agree. I'm still so very hurt and angry sometimes. On a good day, I am able to pray for those people. Other days, I am indifferent. But Christianity is not a religion of indifference. We are called to love and pray for those who have hurt us. Christ was able to do this. I fight to do this, too, but it's a long and wearying battle that ends more often in defeat than victory.

I travel through time when I visit the church of my youth. So much is the same—the pews, the carpet, the hymnals. I open one and my fingers find familiar favorites, those hymns that carried me through the darkness. I spend most of the service staring at that stained glass window from St. Mark's gospel where Jesus, haloed by the sun, gathers the children unto himself. It is a precious grace that I do not hold Him responsible for the sins of those who claimed His name, but I think I will never understand what it feels like to be truly loved or valued in this lifetime, by Him or others. I wonder what I would be like if I had not been raped. Would I be able to feel God's love for me? Would I still feel compassion for broken people? Would I be married? Would I have children? I wonder what might have been. I wonder what will be.

The future stretches before me in dim uncertainty. Brokenness is all I have known, and there is a sense of safety in the familiar. Even though I pursue healing, even though I want it and need it, it can still be scary sometimes. Questions linger. Will I always struggle with PTSD? Will I ever overcome the sense of worthlessness that haunts me? Will I ever be able to reach the frightened little girl I was and convince her that she is safe? I don't know. Perhaps I will. I hope I will. I am certainly trying. But the truth is, we do not always find complete healing in this life. Sometimes, we bear our burdens and find instead that His grace is sufficient. I don't have the answers I want, but in all things, He remains, and He is where I find my ultimate hope. My life will never be what it might have been, but He will provide for me where I am. All shall be well.

I think about heaven a lot, especially the final heaven, when the world is renewed and made whole once again. I don't want mansions and cities and crowns and all the other flashy rewards spoken of in Scripture. I want only Him. I picture my own little cottage on the edge of a forest, big enough for me and my cats and one visitor at a time, because you can't really talk when you're in a group. Sometimes, that visitor is a friend. Most of the time, it's Jesus. And though I fight the familiar battle—*He would never visit me. He'll be too busy with everyone else*—it's a wonderful place. The breeze carries the laughter of children. There's no more violence. No more fear. Nothing negative invades that space. There is only light and love and every good thing.

No one ever asks to be visited by the horrors of life. I would like to think that I'm the only one who has such things as will not let go, that others who have been raped as children have been able to experience total healing. On the chance that I am not alone in this, however—on the chance that there are others who know too well the stubborn, lingering effects of PTSD that spring from childhood sexual assault—I write this so that when you read it, you will know that you are not alone. Much love to you, dear ones.

AM I A WHOLE PERSON?

BY ANONYMOUS

I am a whole person—soul, mind, and body. And I am a follower of Jesus Christ.

But after a forty-five-minute sermon at my church last winter, I felt like a very poor representation of personhood and of Christ.

The pastor had spoken on the topic of anxiety that morning. He had some solid points about the value of training our minds to focus on things other than worst case scenarios, even bringing up Cognitive Behavioral Therapy, a technique I've used often.

But I had some challenges with what he shared from the pulpit too. He also said there was no need for medication in the life of a Christian. He urged those of us who use medications to reevaluate, to quit concentrating on our anxiety in favor of inviting Jesus into our anxiety so He could heal it.

When I left church that morning, I felt less-than. Lazy. Faithless. I felt as though I'd failed.

Let me tell you a little about myself. I am a woman who daily goes to battle with anxiety. This has been my reality every day since I was about eleven years old. Even though I've prayed for healing every moment since, even though others have laid hands on me and prayed for healing, and even though I've memorized every "be strong and courageous" and "do not worry" verse in the Bible, anxiety remains a piece of my life. It still strikes at the most inopportune moments of my life, rendering me a quivering, terrified person frozen in fear.

But Jesus has not been excluded and shoved out of my anxiety.

He's not waiting to engage with my mental health struggles like an old friend waiting for a wedding invitation.

No, I've never even needed to invite Jesus into my battles. He's always been there. Before I knew anxiety, I knew Jesus. I've followed Him since I was a very young child. To speak with complete candor, if Jesus had not firmly planted Himself right in the middle of my battle with anxiety, I would not be here to talk about my battles at all.

Sometimes He acts in ways I can see. I have a mental picture of Jesus wielding a fiery sword of truth and justice, slicing through and decapitating the darkness that lingers. That's my favorite, when we battle together and the heavy talons of anxiety fall around our feet, shriveled up and dying.

But then there are also many times when I've been laid flat out on the bathroom floor, heart racing, feeling like I'm going to choke or throw up or die or all three at once. When there is no fighting, only the words from a repetitive worship song reverberating through my soul while my mind and body quake: "You're a good, good Father. It's who You are. It's who You are".

He's there, too.

Jesus is welcome and necessary in my battle. He is also compassionate in my fear. My soul resonates with his nearness, even in the hardest, most terrifying moments of my anxiety.

But it's not only my soul that was impacted. *All* of my personhood—my soul, my mind, and my body—bears witness to the brokenness of the world.

My mind was deeply shaped by a series of traumatic events in my past. It's no surprise, then, that it also built some pretty incredible coping mechanisms to deal with those events. They served me during those times of extreme pain, but I don't need them to serve me anymore. That danger has passed. The pathways are still there, though; they are deep, they seem safe, and they are easy.

It's hard work to fill those ruts in with fresh dirt and new strategies, and it requires all of my concentration sometimes. But that hard work with good counselors has been a blessing to me and to my mind.

My body was also deeply affected by trauma. It holds tightly to the aftereffects in ways I'm not sure I'll ever understand. Though I know it doesn't work this way for everyone, I'm relieved to have found a medication that tones down the terror, softening it by a few decibels, just enough to allow me to put my mind's resources to work. Just enough to keep me fighting well.

I can't treat my soul with medication. That's Jesus's work. But I can treat my body with it, and thankfully, that makes a difference for me.

Thinking about that Sunday now, I have to assume the pastor didn't intend to minimize my pain or the reality of my situation with his sermon. In fact, if we were having a conversation about anxiety as friends at Starbucks, I'm positive his words would be laced with kindness, grace, and empathy. I trust this pastor has put a lot of time and prayer into his journey as a pastor, and into each sermon he preaches. But even pastors misspeak sometimes, and I'm sure they say things that don't convey their hearts as truly as they would like.

When the pastor said we needed to invite Jesus into our anxiety, I think I understand what he meant. He was trying to say that we will never have the truest sense of healing and wholeness without Jesus. And I agree with that, because I believe Jesus did come to offer healing and wholeness to heartsick and broken people like me. Like all of us.

Nevertheless, because he misspoke on the topic of anxiety, I had lots of new and heavy questions tumbling around in my mind that morning after church. I left wondering if anyone in that building was willing to *be the church* to me or would everyone there would simply tell me I needed to let go of the anxiety and focus on Jesus instead.

Would anyone there be okay as a with-er instead of as a fix-er? Was there anyone in church willing to be patient and gentle and near to me the way Jesus is, even in the midst of my real or imagined catastrophes?

Would anybody in church still respect me as a whole person, even if they knew the depth of this singular pain point in my life? Could others in the church sit with people like me in our overwhelmed moments, offering a shoulder instead of a to-do list?

It took several weeks of engaging with these questions before I determined I had a few options.

I could email the pastor with anger clouding my eyes. I could rail against him and tell him how it felt for my anxiety disorder to be packed up and labeled as "Something You Haven't Truly Given to God Because If You Had It Wouldn't Be an Ongoing Hardship." I could leave the church because of this sermon and because of how I felt leaving the sanctuary that day.

Or I could ask for a conversation. I could seek to understand his perspective and offer him some insight into mine. I actually think this sort of dialogue would be welcomed at my church. But a lot of time had passed, and I didn't feel particularly tugged in that direction or called to have that discussion.

After I'd wrestled with my questions and sat in the uncertainty and the discomfort, begged God for wisdom and prayed through my options, my personal course of action in this situation became clearer.

I didn't need to wait for the pastor or anyone else at my church to *be the church* to me or to anyone else.

I am already the church.

God didn't excise my ability to love others well from my spirit the moment anxiety descended upon me. Far from it, in fact. Now I'm starting to think that maybe He's uniquely equipped me to do the difficult work of leaning in and being with others in their pain and sorrow and terror because those things aren't scary to me. They're a reality of living. I can minister to my friends who also battle mental health challenges.

I am a follower of Jesus Christ. And I live with the pain and uncertainty of an anxiety disorder. Now I refuse to hide or be ashamed of that pain so my friends in the church and outside of it will know deep in their souls that they aren't alone in their battles either.

I choose to be the church because Jesus has work to do there too, and I am His to use.

Two Things I Learned about the Church in a Psych Ward

by Chris Morris

I recently spent a week in a mental hospital. There. I said it.

Family life had been a bit stressful, work was going well, and my side business was growing. Oh, and I was editing a new book about mental illness. But for the better part of a week, I realized I was not okay in my head.

I had suicidal thoughts, and I wasn't safe to be left alone at my house. A psychiatric ward was the best place for me to recuperate and return to my normal frame of mind.

While I was there, I learned a lot about myself and how fragile my soul really is. I was truly awestruck by the kindness of the nurses and techs in the ward. And I realized how much my perception of personal freedom was shaped by everyday choices we take for granted—like choosing my own food and schedule.

I also learned a lot about the American church.

Most of the people in my wing of the hospital were either literal widows and orphans, or members of a similarly ignored part of society: a grandma forgotten by her family, a young man whose parents had died tragically and left him ill-equipped to deal with the challenges of life, homeless military veterans whose wartime injuries rendered them unemployable, and struggling drug addicts desperate to get clean but struggling to make it happen.

Each of these people felt that nobody cared about them. From what I could tell, they weren't wrong.

No visitors came for anyone but me that week. Most of the other patients didn't receive any incoming phone calls except from social workers. Outgoing calls involved lots of crying and promises to do better—and very few "I love yous." It broke my heart.

We in local churches need to reassess where we spend our resources at a global level, but we also need to do the same individually. We have the opportunity to demonstrate pure and undefiled religion.

MENTAL ILLNESS IS STILL A DIRTY LITTLE SECRET IN THE CHURCH.

I came face-to-face with my own unhealthiness in the psych ward. There's no way to avoid deep introspection when you're lying in bed under suicide watch.

Every day I carefully consider how much to tell people about my week in the hospital. Because, if I'm honest, I have some shame. *I'm a good Christian, so I shouldn't have ended up where I did* (say the lies I've been fed). And I know I'm not alone.

Nobody wants to talk about the facts, but mental illness is rampant in America. Approximately twenty-five percent of people in the country self-identify with, or have been diagnosed with, one or more mental illnesses.

This includes the "easy" mental illnesses like anxiety or depression, but it's not limited to those. PTSD impacts people from every walk of life, not just military veterans. Narcissism is an epidemic in corporate America. Sometimes it's even considered a strategy for success and advancement. As a country, we are not mentally healthy.

And yet, we continue to hear sermons like *Seven Steps to a Successful Life,* at the exclusion of helping families bring their challenges into the light.

Indeed, most pastors in America say they are not comfortable talking about mental illness or being a part of a support system. Those of us in the church who are struggling mentally feel unwelcome because nobody knows what to do with us.

So we dry our tears, stuff our fears, and pretend everything is okay. Or, we leave the church altogether. I know churches can do better, and that's why I'm sharing my story.

Do people with cancer or other life-threatening illnesses attend church and receive emotional support? Every week. It's possible to treat mental illness as normal, because for so many, it is. It's possible to view depression through an accurate lens, rather than as a sin, and to treat anxiety as something deeper than a lack of faith.

CHURCHES CAN BECOME A SAFE HAVEN FOR THE MENTALLY ILL.

My pastor visited me while I was in the psych ward, and what he said to me gave me hope—for my own future and the church as a whole.

"You have too much to live for. Yes, you're depressed right now, but you are still beautifully and wonderfully made. God's not done with you yet. Don't you go leaving us. People in our church need what you've got."

My pastor didn't shy away from me. He visited me and gave me a snippet of hope in a dark place. He knew what to do, and he did it.

I've felt the affirmation of hearing some of my own mental health conditions mentioned in sermons. I've seen groups of believers rally around a suicidal man to affirm his worth, staving off the darkness with love. I have watched as an anxious woman is enveloped in care instead of ridicule.

So, I choose hope. I believe the future will hold powerful moments where the mentally ill feel inclusion, acceptance, and hope.

There's one more thing I believe: no person can achieve all that God has in mind for them when they exist outside a local church body. Mentally ill or otherwise, each of us only becomes the best version of ourselves, the most clear representation of Jesus, living the most sanctified lives, and expressing the fullness of what God has placed into our hearts—together.

It's time to stop withholding this opportunity for maturity from those with mental illnesses. No more should the lie be told that only the mentally *well* can serve God and pursue Him wholeheartedly. With the exception of Jesus, God has only used broken humans to accomplish his purposes.

ARE YOU OKAY?

Have you ever felt "not okay" in your head? Most have at one time. Instead of running from the reality or shaming yourself, will you bring your thoughts and feelings to God?

The church won't get any better at caring for the mentally ill if we don't talk about it. We need to engage in honest conversations around what mental illness looks like—and welcome people to bring their thoughts and feelings to us.

That's when real change will start. The time is now.

I'm Tired of Wearing a Mask

by Anne Peterson

"Watch me, Dad," Jessica called out, as her twelve-year-old body dove off the pool's edge.

She didn't even have to ask. Mike's eyes were always watching to see what wonderful thing she would do next. That's the kind of dad she has. Soon after, she left the pool.

In minutes, we were home. I loved the fact we had a pool right in our subdivision.

Walking down the hallway, I saw a note taped to our bedroom door.

"Don't wake me up," the note read.

Turning the knob, I expected to hear my husband snoring, so I was surprised to see him crawling on the floor.

"What are you *doing*?" I asked, watching him get up.

He stumbled and fell against the blinds.

The bottle of his pills sat on the dresser.

"Mike! Did you take extra pills?"

His voice was muffled as he fell across the bed.

"Nathan, call 9-1-1!" I yelled, running from the bedroom.

I ran back to check on Mike, my heart beating through my chest.

I dialed my friend, telling her what was going on. "Pray," I said, and hung up.

When the ambulance arrived, questions shot at me like bullets.

"Ma'am, do you know how many pills he took?"

"Has he ever done this before?"

"Has he been depressed?"

Nathan called Jessica down to his room and out of the commotion.

As they wheeled Mike outside, I could see neighbors lining up. One we knew from church came up to me.

"Is there anything we can do to help?" she asked.

"Pray," I whispered, meaning it with all my heart.

"Would you like to follow us?" the ambulance attendant asked.

"You can ride with me," the policeman offered.

"No," I responded to both. "I'll be there in a couple minutes."

My emotions were all over the place. I'd like to tell you concern was the main one, but I'd be lying. Anger was the clear winner.

What was he thinking? How could he do this?

As I entered the lobby of the hospital, I stopped in my tracks.

There sat, not one, but at least five women from my prayer group. They had come to be with me. To lift all of us in prayer.

"Mrs. Peterson, your husband's toxicity levels are extremely high," the doctor said. "If we aren't able to get it under control, we will be forced to medevac him to a hospital in Chicago."

But that's an hour away!

I felt numb inside, as if I were watching the whole scene, not living it. Waiting was excruciating, but knowing there was a group of women praying helped so much. My mind kept trying to envision what our lives would look like without Mike.

No, I told myself, as I pushed those thoughts out of my head.

A short while later, the doctor returned. Miraculously, Mike's levels had stabilized; he was going to be okay. The question remained, would we?

"You can see your husband now," the nurse said.

"Would you like me to go with you?" my pastor asked.

I nodded and we both followed the nurse.

I saw the pastor's mouth moving as he talked with my husband, but I don't remember one word he said.

My husband said something to me, but I could not decipher his words, nor did I want to.

"We'll be moving him into his room. You can follow us if you'd like."

"No!" I blurted out. "I have to get home to my daughter."

I didn't trust myself. I had a feeling if I had stayed, I would have spewed out words that no one should hear.

When I reached the lobby, there were my friends. Women who had prayed with me, just days before at church.

I remember hugging each of them.

I cried the short ride home. Probably cried all night.

I knew my husband struggled with depression. And I wish this was the only time he had made an attempt, but it wasn't. Nor would it be his last. The road ahead would be a long one, and a lonely one, as well.

When a loved one has a physical ailment, it is easier for others to show their concern. When the illness has anything to do with the mind, there is a stigma. It shouldn't be so, but it is.

Even friends who had prayed for us didn't know what to say. It was probably much easier for them to talk to God than to me.

In the days that followed, there was someone who reached out to my husband. Dick was a wonderful man who had struggled with depression himself earlier in his life.

He came to the house, and even if Mike was in bed, he would go in there and tell him, "Come on, let's go for a walk."

Oh, how that ministered to Mike. Oh, how that touched my

heart. It made me feel like we were still approachable, not people who had a sickness that was highly contagious.

There was another woman and her family who also reached out to us after Mike's attempt. They had experienced similar struggles. They knew the pain we were in. When we spent time with them, we felt totally accepted and loved.

But many others stepped away from relationships with us. After a while, when people continually pull back from you, it's just easier to pull back as well. To subtract yourself from social events, to just disappear. After all, you feel invisible anyway.

After Mike's attempt, I still attended church, and I still went to the prayer meetings.

But I felt odd. Possibly because no one else I knew was struggling in this same area.

Mike was not eager to try church again now. Especially knowing people knew about his attempt. Even before that happened, he felt different. I kept wanting to believe that people did care, that they just didn't know how to express it. But he viewed it differently.

"How are you?" someone asked Mike one Sunday.

My husband responded, "Rotten," as I quietly gasped.

The person went on as if my husband said, "I'm fine."

And my husband leaned over and whispered, "See, I told you, no one really cares."

We talked about it later, and I realized this was my husband's perception. To Mike, nobody in the church cared.

I'll never forget that one Saturday at church when they hired a photographer. Our church had decided to update the directory with photos of its members. Each family would receive their own 8x10 portrait.

"Smile," the photographer said. "You're such a beautiful family."

This was just two days after my husband's suicide attempt.

He saw a beautiful family. He didn't know we were all wearing our masks.

Just like the mask my son Nathan wore, years earlier, as a teenager.

"Hello, Anne," I heard as I picked up the phone.

It was Kyle, Nathan's youth leader, but his tone was not the usual.

"What's up, Kyle?"

After a slight pause, Kyle continued, "Anne, I have reason to believe that Nathan is going to hurt himself."

I felt like someone had hit me in the stomach. I was shocked, yes, but it was tinged with anger.

How could this *be happening and I not know? How could* this *be going on in* my *house and I not have a clue?*

When I told my husband, he could not handle it.

I felt so alone. Did I pray? Of course, but I was confused and didn't even know what to pray.

Little did I know that so many were praying right then for our son. People who had invested in him through the youth group. Friends of his he had come to know at church.

I'm certain heaven was quiet as all those people prayed, and one mother let God see her terrified heart.

The phone rang again. I took a deep breath.

"Anne, Nathan's been found. He's okay."

I got off the phone and told Mike and we both cried. Tears of thankfulness, but there were also tears of sadness that my son had made an attempt.

We would come to find out he had also been cutting. When someone cuts, it's because they feel numb. And they create physical pain so they know they are alive.

Church had been there for my son. A couple of friends stayed in contact with me and would ask me how he was.

It would be a long journey. One that included counseling and lots of prayer.

I'm thankful that the youth group and the youth leader were so supportive of Nathan.

With mental illness there is no Band-Aid that fixes everything. And it would be so helpful if people could realize when one family member is ill, the whole family struggles.

Church should be a safe place where people are accepted as they are, with no pretense.

I'm tired of wearing a mask.

An Inconvenient Truth

by Karen deBlieck

I. The Fall

Today I contemplated killing myself.
The shower water ran over me.
What if I slit my wrists?
And the blood streamed down like ribbons.
What sweet release.
It frightened me.
Shook me to my very core
cracking open to release a great moan
and deep sobs from the very depths.
Until I had to sit down under the deluge
because my legs couldn't hold the weight of my grief.
What was the matter with me?
I was happy wasn't I?
A dream job.
A husband who loved me
and would never let me go.
Four beautiful children.
But I felt so incredibly alone.
And raw.
I was disconnected with everything around me.
For so long I had put my feelings in boxes
stacked neatly and safely in my mind.
All my emotions were kept there.

Just like I was taught by my parents—
feelings weren't meant to be shared or expressed.
So I stored them away.
All the hurts and frustrations of my thirty-odd years,
four children, multiple miscarriages, one struggling marriage, my
own heart of unfaithfulness.
And still, I stored it all away.
I laughed it off.
And stored it away.
Until today.
The dam burst
but I'd known there was a leak…hadn't I?
The short fuse with my husband.
My distance from my children.
My avoidance of God.
The need to keep so busy
I had no time to look back at the horrible scars that lay across my
heart.
Or the things I had thrown into the black hole of my mind
where I'd found more and more important information disap-
pearing.
Without my permission.
And so I wept
broken.
And called out to God
the simple plea of my heart.
Why?
And the heavens wouldn't open up.
There were only my tears.

II. GOD'S HOUSE

Me
In a sea of people
The Holy Spirit is moving
Here
In this place
Drawing brothers and sisters in Christ together
    Or so the words from the hymn say
But not me
The waves of the music
The passion
Batter against me like angry waves
In this crowd of people
I am alone
No one knows my pain
No one knows my anguish
God is here
But not with me.
I try to sing
But the words are stuck in my throat
The walls close in
Squeezing a sob from my depths.
I can't stay here
I don't belong
The service finishes
And I run out of the sanctuary
Away from the crowds
I close my eyes
Drawing in the fresh air like a drowning man

I jump
At a hand on my shoulder
"How are you?"
I lick my lips
Thankful my tears have dried.
The ticking of my heart
Shallow beneath my smile.
"Fine."
I am alone.

III. An Inconvenient Truth

Oh,
So you're sad.
I get that way sometimes too.
It will pass.
It's just laziness.
Get up and push yourself forward.
That will get you out of this funk
Pffft
Depression isn't even a thing
If you're truly relying on God
You'll have complete joy.
More prayer
More Bible reading
That'll fix it
Of course you feel lonely
People aren't going to want to be around you if you're such a
downer.

Medication is just a hoax.
This isn't a real sickness.
God's love is enough.
Come out with the ladies' group
What you need is socialization
It must have been something you've done.
Unconfessed sin.
You must repent.
Everyone has problems.
You have to get over yourself.
You're depressed again?
I thought you were over that.
Listen,
I've done everything I can.
Obviously, you aren't willing to put in the work to feel better.

IV. DEVOTION

Breakfast dishes rest in the sink.
Morning light creeps across the hardwood floor.
The house silent after the rush of children
Packing for school.
The tap drips in the kitchen.
A dog huffs on the floor.
I pull my legs up under me
Bible splayed across my lap
In an effort to draw nearer
I must let go
Of the sadness

Of the pain
Of the baggage
Eyes closed
I call out to
Him
Abba
Father
If it is your will…
For a moment there is a flash of my own father in my mind
One I could never please
Although I tried.
I call out again
Abba
Father
But
Now I'm not sure who I am calling to.
Will He answer?
Is there more that I must do?
The words leap from the page
Am I weary enough?
Will the yoke be
too much for me to bear?
Perhaps I am too tiny
Too small
For Him to see
To care
My heart races
Breathing is ragged
Fight or
Flight

I slam the book shut
Tears slide down my face
   He knows the lies in my mind
   How can I face Him?

V. Not Sick

No one comes by
to visit
the phone stays
Silent
No baskets of fruit
Cards of Sympathy
No pans of lasagna
until the kids push their plates away
No offers of childcare
Or house cleaning
Really
It is no surprise
After all
I'm
not
sick

VI. My Dragon

Sitting in the dark
Hair done

Pretty dress on
I am a mess
The sulfur of the invisible beast
steals my breath
My husband's shadow falls across me
"Are you sure you don't want to go?"
I nod my head
I hear him on the phone
"She's not feeling well"
It is
true?
Will I ever feel well again?
He returns
"Anything I can do?"
I shake my head
his shoulders fall
this is one dragon he cannot defeat for me.
He leaves me alone
because sadness deserves to be alone
Although
I wish someone was brave enough
to sit in the darkness
With me
and the beast

VII. PLEASE

See me
when I hide

Invite me
when you know I'll decline
Continue
even when I say stop
Pursue me
as I run
Defend me
from my lying mind
Do not let me
be eaten alive
And
Please
I beg you
Love *me*
when I cannot

VIII. THE FULLNESS OF GOD

Darkness presses in on me
My chains chafe against my raw soul.
Will I ever see the sun again?
Laugh?
A single shaft of light illuminates my mind
  Yes, Jesus loves me
  The Bible tells me so
A simple children's song
Too simple
Too
easy

And yet?

> *Let the little children come to me,*
> *and do not hinder them,*
> *for the kingdom of heaven belongs to such as these.*[3]

Dare I?

I reach out

Tentative

to touch His robes

> *The LORD will fight for you;*
> *you need only to be still.*[4]

But Lord,

I am so weak.

> *I will strengthen you and help you;*
> *I will uphold you with my righteous right hand.*[5]

I tremble.

> *For I am the LORD your God who takes hold of your right hand*
> *and says to you,*
> *Do not fear; I will help you.*[6]

I've tried, LORD, it will not work.

> *Trust in ME with all your heart and lean not on your own*
> *understanding.*[7]

I close my eyes

holding my hands out

"Please free me."

> *Then they cried to the LORD in their trouble,*
> *and he saved them from their distress.*

---

3   NIV Matthew 19:14
4   NIV Exodus 14:14
5   NIV Isaiah 41:10b
6   NIV Isaiah 41:13
7   NIV Proverbs 3:5 (paraphrase my own).

He brought them out of darkness, the utter darkness,
and broke away their chains.[8]

The tears stream down in earnest now.

Darkness clings to me

Loath to let go.

It will always be there

an unwelcome shadow

Even though I walk
through the darkest valley,
I will fear no evil,
for you are with me;
your rod and your staff,
they comfort me.[9]

But His blessing rests over me like

a blanket.

I bow my head to receive it.

I pray that you, being rooted and established in love,
may have power, together with all the Lord's holy people,
to grasp how wide and long and high and deep is the love of
Christ,
and to know this love that surpasses knowledge—
that you may be filled to the measure of all the fullness of God.[10]

So let it surely come to pass.

Amen.

---

8 NIV Psalm 107:13-14
9 NIV Psalm 23:4
10 NIV Ephesians 3:17-19

Stalked by Depression

by Anonymous

I am a Christ-follower, a wife, a mother, a daughter, a sister, an aunt, a friend, a writer, a nurse, and I suffer from a mental illness.

I have been stalked by depression most of my life. I have learned tricks to deal with the depression that help me get through the day. I know when I can handle it on my own and when I need to seek professional help and medication. That doesn't mean I've conquered depression. In fact, that is far from the truth. To make matters worse, the church has been at times helpful and at other times destructive. It's left me feeling confused and untrusting toward any church, as I never know what I am going to hear or receive.

In April of 2007 my depression decided to rear its ugly head in an indisputable way. My third child had been born in March of that year. The older two were three years old and twenty months old. For a woman who never planned on having children, I was overwhelmed. I was trying desperately to squeeze myself into the mold of a "Normal Baptist Woman" and the vision of wife and mother my husband had for me.

My physician noticed during several of visits that I was exhibiting the warning signs of post-partum depression. A kind and caring man, he spent time counseling me and encouraging me to take an antidepressant. I refused his help and denied that I was struggling. I knew I was sad and tired and overwhelmed, but figured all I needed was a good night's sleep. I was wrong. Too deep in its clutches, I was blind to the depth of my depression.

The wakeup call that came still makes me want to put my head down and sob. Most people don't know this piece of my story, but I hope sharing it here will help bring to light how powerful depression can be. I was cutting cheese for my oldest daughter's lunch. She and my son started fighting, then the baby woke up and started crying. I looked at the knife in my hand and thought to myself, "I've had enough. I can't do this. I can't go on." The temptation to end it all right then and there for my three children and myself was so strong that I felt my hand tighten on the knife and I brought it up.

I can only credit God that my children and I are here today. I couldn't move from that spot. A still, small voice whispered to my heart God's love, his understanding, and his strength available to me. He held my hand still, held me tight until a little of his light slipped into the darkness. He whispered to me to put the knife down and call my doctor.

Shaking, I dropped the knife, picked up the phone and called my doctor. Through God's perfect timing, my doctor was available to talk to me. All I had to say was, "I think I need those pills."

My doctor heard and understood but would only give me the pills if I attended counseling. I readily agreed. Guilt was settling in, the same guilt that holds me in its grasp over a decade later. I needed to find a path to better health.

I started taking an antidepressant and found a spiritual counselor. She was just what I needed. She listened to me, she gave me the permission I needed to be the kind of mother and wife God created me to be, and she encouraged me to stop trying to fit into someone else's box. She helped me talk to my husband, who didn't realize the pressure his unconscious expectations put on me.

You may be wondering, what about the church? After all, this is a collection of essays on mental health and the church. Eighteen years ago, I began to attend a Baptist church, my then fiancé's church.

Shortly before I started attending, a new pastor stepped into the leadership role at this church. Under his leadership, I saw the church make a radical shift from being inward-focused to welcoming and community oriented. They even accepted someone off-centered like me. God sent me good friends, who were also a little off-centered and whom I still love dearly.

This pastor also suffered from anxiety and depression. He understood my depression better than most of the congregation, so they took their cues from him. There wasn't a big deal made about my depression

They prayed for me. In church, members inquired how I felt, asked if I needed anything, and let me know they were praying for me. I felt loved and accepted. They never treated me like an outcast or unclean.

My post-partum depression was difficult. It hit unexpectedly and plunged me deep into darkness and despair. But, I resurfaced almost as quickly. I attribute that to not only the medication and counseling, but to the love I received at this Baptist church. For a bout of depression, as I look back on it from the other side, it was a smooth one.

I learned a lot from my first battle with depression. I felt armed and prepared. Although I knew that I would never be free from its presence, I felt capable to battle the darkness and keep it under control.

In the spring of 2014, the perfect storm occurred and drowned me in depression again. A combination of not sleeping well for months and consuming large amounts of sugar and caffeine sent my heart into SVT (Super Ventricular Tachycardia). My heart raced close to three hundred beats per minute for almost an hour, which equates to running a 5K in five minutes. Exhausted, I slept for several days afterwards. I did not realize my depression and physical difficulties fed into each other in a vicious cycle. I still do not know which issue came first, just that they caused a downward spiral into darkness.

I worked for months to medically fix the physical causes, but I found I still didn't feel right. Sleep eluded me. My energy was so low, I'm not sure how I made it through even one day without collapsing. I wore a halter monitor for two days to watch my heart. I spent the night in a sleep lab checking for sleep apnea. Tubes of blood were taken for every test my provider could think of. Everything came back normal.

The nurse practitioner treating me at the time sat me down after all the testing. She explained that she believed me when I did not feel right, but she found nothing medically wrong. She believed my physical problems were manifestations of a new episode of major depression and prescribed Ativan to help me sleep and Lexapro for my depression. She also encouraged me to seek alternate therapies. Despite the lessons of the past, I yet again denied that I was in the grip of depression.

I denied it for several more months. It wasn't until I decided it might be a good idea to take the whole bottle of Ativan and the whole bottle of Lexapro that I truly recognized depression's return. Thankfully, I had a good friend I could turn to. She made sure to get those pills from me without any hint of judgment.

God also directed me to a group of alternate nutritionists, whom I still see today. Supplements and a proper diet are used to help control both physical and psychological issues. It's not a quick fix, and I struggle to follow the guidelines. When I do eat right, I feel better and it is easier to control my depression.

At home and work, I was doing better controlling my depression, slowly digging myself out of the miry muck I had unwittingly buried myself in. After months and months of struggle, I finally started to see glimpses of light. But, no matter what I did, I was trapped there, balanced between darkness and light, fighting hard to keep the little light I had.

It was frustrating to be unable to make forward progress, no matter what I tried. Several times I thought about giving up, just letting the depression suck me back in and to stop fighting.

Early in November of last year, the struggle finally tipped in my favor. I started to chip away large chunks of darkness to bring in more light. As I look back, I realize the change that tipped the scale was one God had been calling me to do for over a year. The change was not something I could have done on my own; it also involved my family.

We left the Baptist church I had been a member of for over eighteen years. I can't blame them for the depression I suffered, but I believe it is because of that church that the depression lasted as long as it did. I knew going to church and interacting with the people there caused my anxiety to increase, which in turn fueled my depression. At first, I wasn't sure why that would be. It wasn't the first time I had a major depressive experience while attending there.

When my crisis first appeared, I pulled out of everything at church. Just attending on a Sunday morning was a weekly struggle. At first, the members of the church provided the same care as before. Unfortunately, that would change.

Some churches morph to fit the personality of their pastor. This Baptist church is one of them. Many members who once supported me through my post-partum depression were still in the church, but their view of me and how they treated me changed. I don't know what they believed about my second round of major depression, but the love and care shown previously disappeared.

I could go months without anyone speaking to me, other than a brief good morning. Even when I openly wept in my pew, no one said anything. No one came to me and asked why I wasn't getting involved and no one visited. Maybe the concern was there, it just wasn't expressed.

Looking back, with a clearer mind, I can point to three other things that differed between the first and second episodes. All three of these factors are interconnected and served to create a feeding ground for my depression. All three differences centered on the church I had been attending at the time. Even though it was the same church, my experience was dramatically different between the two bouts of depression for several reasons. First, many of my close friends and supporters moved out of the area. I didn't have anyone safe to be real with. Instead I had to decide to either put my "Normal Baptist Woman" mask on and fake it entirely, or risk being exposed with nobody to shield me.

Second, I suffered from a different type of depression the second time around. I often wonder if the way I was treated the second time had to do with the type of depression I experienced. Post-partum depression has a very obvious cause—giving birth. It is often self-limiting. Based mostly on hormonal changes, it is considered by many to be a physical disease, not a mental illness. In other words, post-partum depression was acceptable, but major depressive episodes were not.

But the biggest difference was that there was a new lead pastor. When my depression began to spiral out of control, my husband and several friends advised me to seek counseling. They all recommended I see this new pastor.

I had my doubts about seeing the new pastor. During the year he had been pastoring the church, I had noticed things he said or did that bothered me. I also knew from my past experience with depression and counseling that you have to be willing to open yourself up to the counselor. Just like there are people you click with and become friends with and some you don't, the same can be said for counselors. But my husband and friends kept encouraging me, so my husband and I began meeting with him.

At first, things seemed to be going okay. We had some of the same interests in nerdy TV shows and movies, had read some of the same books, and he seemed to have respect for my slightly off-center views on life. Then little things started to creep in, little things I didn't agree with but that weren't all that important. Little things like telling me to stop reading, watching, and writing about fantasy or sci-fi; to stop listening to friends who were free-spirited; and to avoid contact with the Christians involved with the writers' conference I attended.

Supposedly all of these contributed to my anxiety and depression by placing bad thoughts and ideas in my head. Those little things started to add up, plus bigger issues began to surface. I felt under attack and wanted to stop the sessions, but my husband requested I try just a little more. He believed the new pastor was just trying to understand me. Sadly, this was only the beginning of a dark turn in my counseling sessions with the pastor.

So, I continued, but with a change. I went to counseling with the idea that he was unable to help me because he didn't understand me. I decided I would have to help him understand me first, so then he in turn could help me. I found this delightful book, *Introverts in the Church* by Adam S. McHugh. I highlighted passages that I felt would help the new pastor better understand me. While he had heard of the differences between introverts and extroverts, and would himself be classified as an introvert, he stated he didn't really believe in it.

He saw no reason to make allowances for someone who liked quiet moments during worship services and would never include them in his services. Further, he said that supposedly introverted people would have to be mature in their faith and adapt to how the church was being run. He told me these things in our counseling session, despite the fact that he often would state publicly that there were many forms of worshiping God. It became obvious he didn't actually believe those words.

I became hurt and angry with him and my husband grew more uncomfortable with what was being said to me and how the new pastor was treating me. I decided to maintain the counselee role, but used silence to see what happened. What I learned did not surprise me, it only made me angry and sad.

As a nurse and a Christian, I have studied science, medicine, and the Bible. I fully believe that there can be both physical and spiritual influences that contribute to mental health diseases. I believe failure to recognize this fact leads to imperfect treatment by both sides. Medicine tends to focus only on treating the physical, while religions tend to focus only on the spiritual. It is only when we bring the two together that a person can truly begin to heal.

That was not the new pastor's view. After almost a year of meeting with him, his true views on mental illnesses came to light. At this point, I was out of the deepest part of my depression, but still struggled to completely move past the depression. My forward progress was a slow struggle. The pastor was unsatisfied at my pace and seemed to feel I should have thrown off my depression fully by now.

As I mentioned, I began to use silence to see where he was going with his questions. We had been talking about the fruit of the Spirit. He had supplied a piece of paper with an image on it of a tree and its roots. The fruit of the Spirit was already labeled in the tree. The pastor asked me to fill in the roots with which I nourished my tree. Fair enough. I started entering those things I believed would be needed to have a healthy, fruitful life.

He was unhappy with my roots. Unsure why he was unhappy, I kept silent. That's when he hit me with it.

"Depression is only caused by deep-rooted, horrible, secret sins. And until you confess those sins you will continue to have depression. I think it's a good time for you tell me what those sins are."

My husband, sitting next to me, and I just stared at him for a few moments. I wasn't sure how to respond at first. I wanted to remain calm and respectful. My husband said afterwards he expected me to explode.

I didn't explode. I simply asked the pastor about all the research out there showing both chemical and physical changes in the bodies and brains of those with mental illnesses. I even offered to open up my computer and show him articles.

The pastor's response: "There is nothing you can show me that will change my mind on this. Science is lying on this matter and I don't believe scientists know what they are talking about."

As a nurse and as a Christian I was flabbergasted. I couldn't wrap my brain around how someone who enjoyed watching Star Trek and had smart gadgets galore could ignore science in this area. Data is data. It's just there, with nothing to prove.

Thankfully, we were nearing the end of the scheduled counseling time. My husband and I sat in silence. Neither one of us had anything to say. After a few minutes of this, the pastor told me to think about it and asked when we could meet again. I said I wasn't sure, since our schedule was up in the air, but we would let him know.

I never contacted him again about meeting for counseling. Even though we continued to attend the Baptist church for two years, he never once asked how things were going with my depression, nor inquired when I wanted to continue counseling.

In a church that takes its cues and attitudes from the pastor, I saw a vast difference in how I was treated as a person with mental illness. The first pastor was a full supporter of those who suffer, and that showed in the attitudes of the people in the church. The second pastor obviously wasn't. I can't say the members of the church were outright mean in their treatment and words. It was just a quiet shunning, a turning away and a fear of going against the pastor.

We officially left in November of 2017. For years I struggled with and tried to recover from my depression in an increasingly uncaring church. Forcing myself to go every Sunday was agony. Anxiety fed my depression and kept the struggle going for much longer than it would have had I felt the support of the church.

My husband and I spent over a year discussing whether or not we should leave. It's not a decision we made lightly. Finally, after much prayer and discussion with our parents, we decided it would be better to leave.

Several times since we've left, people from the Baptist church have contacted me to say they miss seeing us in our usual seats. Left unspoken are the questions about why we left and when we're coming back. Part of me misses them, but a bigger part wants to write back and ask them where they were when I sat sobbing on Sunday mornings, to ask them why they ignored my withdrawal from everything I had been involved in and my refusal to be involved. Why did they ignore me and my sufferings?

A month after we left, my anxiety lessened dramatically. I can attend church with few issues. I enjoy the singing again and, most of the time, I don't cry. The church we're going to is delightful. The people are welcoming. The pastor makes statements several times a month to the effect that this is the people's church and they decide what to do; he's just there for direction. I like that. Even without knowing about my mental illness, the pastor has spoken about how to treat those who struggle. He acknowledges the mind-spirit connection, the idea that the body can have physical issues that lead to mental health issues, and the need to treat both sides of things. That is very encouraging.

But my husband wants to become a member. He's ready to settle down and be involved again. The kids are happy there and want to stay, even if they miss their old friends. I'm not there yet.

Even thinking about joining the church while writing this causes my anxiety to spike and the depression starts to ooze into the edges of my brain. My fight or flight reaction kicks in and tells me to run, to attend a different church, to church hop.

Even the thought of going there permanently without being a member scares me. I can keep up the pretense of being normal for now, for the short term. Becoming a member, or even going long term, means becoming involved and building relationships with people. A good church won't accept anything less.

I can maintain the façade of normality only as long as I can keep myself apart, stick to brief small talk, and avoid too many deep interactions with my fellow believers. In this church, it's not possible to do that. They already are seeking me out and asking more than what I can give.

I'm at a loss for what to do. I'm still so wounded by the lies my previous pastor told me about mental illness. I'm stuck. This is what being mentally ill in the church has done to me—I'm afraid to be in church now.

Intellectually, I know God has called me into Christian community and part of me misses that kind of fellowship and life. But the idea of having to start over yet again, to go through that whole process is exhausting to think about, disheartening, and scary. I struggle to trust anyone. I'm panicking as I write this. My heart is starting to race, tears are coming to my eyes, and my feet feel the urge to move, to escape. Dread settles in to squeeze my heart.

I just can't.

A Realm of Hope

by Josh Hardt

Let me start out by saying I love the churches I've been involved with. But to say that they're great at meeting the needs of those with mental illnesses would be a falsehood. It would be easy to tell you about my poor experiences in that regard. Instead, I'm going to tell you about how a group of rebels, misfits, and dreamers saved my life.

Cue flashback.

Back in 2014, I'd learned about the Realm Makers writers' conference from several of my author friends. Realm Makers is a conference for speculative fiction writers of faith. Spec fic, as we like to call it, is where all the "weird fiction" belongs—fantasy, science fiction, horror, and the like.

It seemed like a good move for a fledgling author, so I made the trek to St. Louis the following July. It was amazing, and suffice it to say that I could gush about how awesome it was for several thousand words. The part that matters for this story, though, is what I found there.

Never outside of my marriage had I experienced the level of acceptance I experienced at Realm Makers. No church, campus organization, or friendship I'd previously experienced could match the instant acceptance I found there.

It didn't matter that I was weird and twitchy. No one cared when I laughed a little too loudly. These people that I'd built relationships with online didn't flinch. Frankly, I'm still surprised.

But there's more to this story...

I left the conference with more than a few new siblings-in-Christ. In the weeks that followed, I got to know and build trust with several of them. Then, as it often goes, a God thing happened:

"Have you thought that you might be autistic, Josh?"

This came from two of these trusted siblings in the same day. No mean-spirited attitude came with the question. Just curiosity and honest concern. After talking with my wife and some of my closest advisors, and after a lot of prayerful consideration, I decided to go in for testing. There could be a whole separate treatise on just how much of a headache that whole process was.

The day of the testing came quicker than expected. Sooner than I'd wanted. But here we were. My wife and I traveled to the testing facility. The questions went on for hours. I was asked everything from how much water I drink to how often I've contemplated suicide. Some of the questions made me flinch and wonder how screwed up I really was. Three hours later, it was done. We'd soon have answers we'd been seeking for a long time.

Four days later, life changed forever. Autism. Anxiety. Depression. ADHD. A quartet of neurosensory disorders to call my very own.

How can I explain what I felt without pulling out the melodramatic adjectives? Numb and tired, maybe. There was an emptiness I hadn't ever experienced before. For a few days I was little more than an organic logic machine. That didn't last for long, with so much emotion bubbling beneath the surface.

See, there's a cycle of grief that goes with being diagnosed with a chronic illness. Mine was something close to the classic five stages (denial, then anger, then bargaining, then depression, and finally acceptance), but I had bonus constant companions of guilt and bitterness.

Guilt that I would never be able to be a fully functional husband and father. Shame that I'd inadvertently damaged previous relationships I couldn't get back. Bitterness at the realization that there would be times I wouldn't be able take care of myself, let alone anyone else.

The self-loathing and depression? There's no describing that without getting a little theological. It was emotional hell. Nothing could shake me from the funk. Instead it fed on itself and my hope, sending me into a downward spiral.

On a good day, I could go through the motions. Those rare exceptional days I'd even manage a genuine laugh. And I was quite good at pretending everything was okay during those times. Usually, though, I yelled. At God, myself, my family...really whoever sought to comfort me. When I wasn't bellowing I was bitterly remarking about my poor lot in life.

Despite my moments of lucidity, it didn't take me long to decide I wasn't worth much at all. Who was I, this pathetic little broken thing, to intrude upon everyone else? I'd had bad stretches before I was diagnosed, sure, but nothing like this.

Even on a good day, when I was in love with the rest of the world, there was no reason to consider myself worthwhile. Even when I was worshipping God or having fun with my family and friends, there was a barrier between me and joy.

As it turns out, God loves us entirely too much to allow such nonsense for long. You see, even when flailing ineffectually at these demons I had crowding around me, God was talking to the people who loved me. Then it came, the question that would end up saving my life.

"You going to Realm Makers this year?"

Friends asked me. Family inquired. People I hardly knew except through author friends asked me. Now, I was still playing the "everything's fine" game. I was doing a damn good job of it, too. I made sure to keep off video messaging as much as possible with those who knew me well. Work stress was the excuse I gave to cover the rest. My wife and children were about the only people I couldn't fool. Nor was I stupid enough to try.

Beneath this façade, I was fading. Even when I was giggling with my family and chilling with friends, I had a growing sense that none of it mattered. Yes, I'd made plans to go to Realm Makers, but it didn't change the bedrock truth I knew in the core of my being—*I didn't matter.*

This essay isn't about the finer points of spiritual warfare. But make no mistake, it's something every person who deals with a long-term or chronic illness encounters. And the church has enough trouble deciding what to say about combating spiritual reality without throwing sickness into the mix. Where in the world was I going to turn? I was a jumbled mess of despairing messages and hopeful refrains from those who cared about me.

Truth was, for every person who voiced love, there was opposition in my head. Thoughts tumbled out, unwanted but unwavering. Taunting the very idea of hope, telling me that I didn't deserve anything positive because I was damaged goods.

"Sure, you're loved. But why? Not like you're worth it."

"Look at you, laughing with your family. You don't deserve happiness."

But these people in my life kept asking questions. Sometimes it was about Realm Makers or my writing journey. Others about that new movie or video game. No matter the question, I began to hear what they were really saying.

"We love you, Josh."

I could probably stop there and let it be enough. After all, I'm obviously still here. There's more, though.

I'm sitting here writing these words, and I'm dry-eyed but shaking. These next words aren't easy to type. But they're true.

I made my plans to go to Realm Makers. I held my loved ones close, including my new Realm Makers friends, with a ferocity borne of desperation. And then I decided that I'd end my life once I knew whether my novel-in-progress would net me a contract.

Strange as it sounds, I was relaxed after I'd made the decision. I had maybe a year to go until the struggle was over. So why worry about it anymore? I enjoyed the flight to St. Louis en route to Realm Makers in Reno. I was even starting to look forward to the trip.

And yet again I underestimated God.

In St. Louis, author friends I'd only met over the internet joined me on the plane. And there it was. That same love that had come from words on a screen was hovering there around these people. And it was directed toward me. Me! The one who was too broken to deserve any such thing!

The East Coaster who I barely knew? Joy that was near palpable. And quite infectious. The marketing manager whom I'd exchanged a *single* email with years prior? Unnecessary patience. The shuttle full of tired travelers? Quiet assurance.

And all of that was before we'd even hit the conference proper.

Then it was the sister-in-love who clotheslined me with a hug. The people working the desk who broke into genuine smiles of delight when they saw me. And the others—so many others—who I knew dealt with their own illnesses but still chose to pray with and for me.

So what's my point?

It was a bunch of guys wearing Captain America shirts, not a suit-and-tie-wearing Sunday school leader that proved to me I was worthwhile after all.

It was a group of friends making silly faces and speaking in ridiculous accents around a game of Superfight! that finally cracked the wall that was separating me from experiencing happiness.

And it was an overworked and exhausted conference director that, because she took the time to listen, allowed me to finally cry about my circumstances.

The geeks and misfits I know, whether in the same room as me or halfway across the world, are the church I belong to. And they rescued me from despair, hopelessness, and suicide. They have a lot of wisdom and even more *agape*. Even if it is interrupted by geeky quotes from sci-fi shows like *Firefly* and *Star Trek*.

Jesus Holds Me Together

by Heather Cook

My name is Heather and I struggle with Post Traumatic Stress Disorder or PTSD. PTSD looks different for each person suffering from it. It's a very internal and personal battle. The suffering is difficult to share, because I don't want to be a burden on others.

Truth is, Jesus Christ is the only reason I've made it this far. He's the glue that holds me together and makes me whole.

I've done everything I can to seem normal in the past. I could have been the person sitting next to you, looking like I have everything together. That's how Christians are supposed to look, right? I rehearsed small talk in my head just in case a well-meaning person approached me. I adjusted my mask to make sure nobody could see the mess behind it. This mask I wore every day was heavy, but I was terrified to remove it.

I was afraid of what you might think if you only knew the truth about what went on inside me. I feared you'd question my devotion to Jesus Christ and your judgment is more than I could bear. So, the mask stayed on most days. I told myself that my pain is mine alone; there's no way I would ever wish this upon anyone else.

But today, I'm going to invite you into my mess, into my PTSD.

I imagine my memories would look very much like a dusty old attic. In one corner is my little tea set, daintily set up on my tiny table with my dolls awaiting tea. In another corner is my toy kitchenette where I'd mix my mother's various lotions and sprays, making magic potions I imagined could do wondrous things. My graduation cap and gown hang on a dusty old coat rack.

Alongside the sweet and innocent memories are monsters lurking in the shadows, ready to jump out and devour me. Sifting through the happy memories often leads to the ones I wish I could forget. It wasn't one traumatic event that led to my PTSD, but many events led to this constant reality in my life.

As a small child, my babysitter used me to produce child pornography. I didn't even have control of what happened to my own body. In my adolescence I experienced intense and pervasive bullying, and I couldn't even escape it in my own home. Dysfunction surrounded me daily and everything was beyond my control.

I taught myself to suppress those awful memories and the associated emotions. Eventually, I became adept at suppressing everything. I was numb. In addition to suppressing my emotions, I began to hurt myself in a multitude of ways. Self-harm was the only way I could feel anything at all, starting with a safety pin at ten years old. I was careful not to allow anyone to see what I was doing.

I didn't even realize how numb I had become until one of my closest childhood friends passed away. I remember seeing people distraught with grief at the funeral home but I couldn't muster a tear. I looked around and wondered, "What's wrong with me? Why don't I feel anything?" Unbeknownst to me, I was already struggling with PTSD at the age of fifteen.

Would it surprise you that I was first introduced to Jesus Christ during those tender years?

I wish I could say my experience with church in my childhood was great, but I'd be lying. It had good moments. I loved going to vacation Bible school with my neighbors, and going to church with my best friend was always a welcome reprieve from the chaos swirling inside my home.

Of course, my parents wanted nothing to do with church. I remember people from church coming to my house, claiming to just be in the neighborhood, and inviting my parents to visit. My parents would become angry; I was always the kid whose parents didn't attend.

To make matters worse, I didn't have nice clothes and usually wore whatever was clean. I wasn't the type of girl that liked to wear dresses anyway. As I grew up and continued to attend, the way I dressed became an issue.

I remember asking, "Wouldn't God want us to be with Him no matter how we're dressed?" The question was not received well. Instead of compassion, I only received anger and indignation.

"Stop asking questions; that's just the way it is. If you can't dress nice in your Father's house, then you shouldn't come at all."

I never went back.

If that Sunday school teacher knew what was going on in my life rather than simply passing judgment upon me, maybe my walk with Christ would have gone differently. Maybe I wouldn't have gone down such a dark and disturbing path. But she didn't. I started reading the books my mother was giving me about witchcraft. I ran from the judgment of the church and straight into the occult.

Witchcraft became my addiction. It was appealing because I spent most of my life without control and witchcraft provided me an illusion of power. I thought I could direct the world around me, but it turned out, darkness began controlling me instead. I would spend the next seventeen years chasing this delusion.

In 2007, God reached out and plucked me from my proverbial prison with a dramatic and humbling conversion. After choosing to follow Christ, I lost the vast majority of my friends, and some of my former friends became hostile toward me. Considering most of my friends were pagan, I suppose it's understandable that darkness would flee from the light. That didn't make it hurt any less. It was God's provision that my family and I moved to the same county where I grew up.

Returning to church wasn't easy. I was always an outsider at the church from my childhood, and my past was sordid, haunting me everywhere I went. I would get up early on Sunday and research churches, trying to choose one to attend, but the thought of returning conjured anxiety. I could never choose, so I ended up going nowhere.

Then a woman at my sons' bus stop invited me to her church. An invitation is what I needed—I was all too happy to join her. But I was in no way prepared for what I experienced in that sanctuary. This church was more charismatic than what I knew as a child, and it made me uncomfortable. My anxiety was heightened when at the end of service, my new friend dragged me to the front to pray.

I remember looking up at the cross and feeling genuine sorrow for my past but an inescapable panic overwhelmed me. At the foot of the cross, I could no longer hide behind my mask. But this church was not for me.

The next Sunday I loaded up my children and drove twenty miles to the only church I remember ever feeling welcome, New Hope Christian Church. I still tried to hide behind a mask, not allowing anyone to know the real me. As far as they knew, I grew up in a Christian home and loved Christ my entire life. Façades only last so long.

One Sunday, without warning, I found myself confessing my history with the occult to my Sunday school class. I poured out my sins in a torrent of tears and sobs. I expected judgment, but instead was met with compassion.

I attended New Hope for years and developed several friendships. I live over three hundred miles away now but I still visit whenever I am able. They were my first church family. Although I felt welcome, I was still wearing a mask. I remained numb from my PTSD, but on occasion, my exterior would crack and a glimpse of the chaos inside crept out. I hid darker secrets, but so long as I looked the part of the good Christian, nobody questioned otherwise.

In 2016 my family moved to middle Tennessee and my first goal was to find a church home. I visited a few and began attending a very large church with a beautiful and ornate building. It was lovely and the people matched. I again found myself playing a part and keeping up the appearance of a good Christian. I attended regularly and joined the Wednesday morning moms' Bible study. I began to cultivate relationships with the other women.

When I joined the women's Bible study, they were nearly done working through a book I had already studied, so I felt confident in sharing during discussion. A few weeks before the book was done, the leader announced the next study. It just so happened to be a study about spiritual warfare, something I knew all too well. Having been pagan in the past, I felt it was necessary to make my group leader aware.

In private, she told me my experiences could frighten others in the group and asked me to keep my sharing within the Holy

Spirit's leading. I wish I could say I was able to provide valuable insight for the study, but I wasn't able to contribute much at all. My group leader would begin talking over me whenever I tried to share.

Eventually, I stopped trying. In a room full of seventy-five women, I felt alone and judged.

I asked the leader if she or other women would like to do a more in-depth study. She said no, but suggested a few people; those few people passed me to others, who passed me to others. It wasn't long before I began to feel unwelcome and cast aside. I stopped attending the church, and nobody seemed to notice. Only one person contacted me two months later, asking if I planned to return or if she could take me off the email list. So, my search for a church started again.

The search ended a few weeks later. My family doesn't celebrate Halloween, but we did attend several different trunk-or-treat events. One of them was at The Experience Community.

There were tons of happy kids and parents stuffed into a parking lot, cars lined up with smiling people handing out candy. Batman and a few of his colleagues even showed up. Several people manned the grill, handing out free hotdogs. One woman frantically cleaned the tables.

My teenage sons were complaining about boredom, so I suggested they help clean tables. The relief on the woman's face when my sons started helping was enough to send me into action. I started cleaning up too. Suddenly, she began talking to me like I'd been attending the church for years.

The next Sunday morning, I visited The Experience. I was taken aback by the condition of the building. It was very old. The roof leaked in places and the ceiling rafters were in plain view.

It was a far cry from the vast and magnificent sanctuary I called home only a month prior. On the walls were beautiful pieces of art, created in worship of our Heavenly Father.

Many would look at this building as something to be demolished and rebuilt, but I found it inspiring. For me, the building itself was a massive reminder of humanity's status: broken, beautiful, and so very loved. I felt at home.

I dove in headfirst and checked out several groups before I attended the membership class, called Next. This night opened my heart in many ways. Corey Trimble, the pastor of The Experience, gave his testimony, and for the first time, I not only respected and admired my pastor—I identified with him. His story wasn't so different from mine. He faced his brokenness, owned it, and turned it over to Christ. He didn't hide from it. He was real. I wanted the same.

I became involved with Celebrate Recovery. It surprised me that Celebrate Recovery wasn't just for addictions. It addresses addiction but can target any hurt, habit, or hang-up that prevents you from living the full life God intends. In February 2017, I revealed the darkest secrets of my childhood.

I said aloud what happened to me in the safety of my abuse group. I revealed that my babysitter sexually abused me and took pictures while doing so. Not only that, men would come to the house to either watch or participate. Thirty years of hiding behind masks ended that night. The greatest stronghold Satan had over me fell and a rush of warmth filled the room.

Shortly after that night, I began a Christian 12-step program and started seeing a Christian therapist. I didn't know I had been suffering from PTSD for nearly thirty years. I thought PTSD was characterized only by flashbacks and triggers. But for me, it manifested as emotional numbing. Without The Experience, Corey's testimony, and Celebrate Recovery, I'd still be emotionally paralyzed.

What was it about The Experience that made all this possible? They're not afraid of getting their hands dirty. They meet people where they are, right in the middle of their messes. They feed the homeless every weekend. They hand out hotdogs to people leaving bars after a night of drinking, sometimes putting them in cabs and paying the fares—no questions asked and more importantly, no judgment.

The most important aspect of The Experience and their ability to reach those who suffer is their authenticity. They do not shy away from their own histories of brokenness. Whether they have struggled with drugs, pornography, self-harm, mental illness, or anything; they're not afraid to be real. It just takes one person to step forward and reveal their struggle, creating a ripple effect. It inspires courage in others to face their own brokenness.

I'm still learning to be real. I'm nearly forty years old, and for the first time, I'm getting to know who I am. I've worn masks for so long, I lost who God created me to be. My slate is clean and my heart made of clay, ready to be formed by my loving Savior. Real changes have happened in my life. As of April 2018, I'm one year sober from self-harm.

What He plans to do and where He intends to take me is yet to be seen. The freedom I experience now is indescribable in comparison to the prison I created for myself. How can I not want to share? This freedom is available to everyone, even the mentally ill. Especially the mentally ill, perhaps.

Jesus Christ is the best answer to combat mental illness, but all too often, those struggling are shunned by the church. What are we afraid of? Maybe it's time we all take a look in the mirror, remove the masks, and face our own brokenness.

We're all broken somehow. God never intended the church to be a sanctuary of saints. Jesus Christ is the Great Physician and His church is a hospital for the broken.

Coming to the End to Find My Beginning

BY JAMES PRESCOTT

When you tell a story of mental illness, it's not like any other story. Most stories have a beginning, a middle, and an end. An end which can sometimes be happy, sometimes tragic, others melancholy. But an end, nonetheless.

Mental health stories aren't quite the same.

Those of us with some kind of mental illness know this of our own stories. Because mental illness isn't something to be cured. It's part of our wiring, it's how our brains work. It's part of us, every single day—the only thing we can change is how we live with it, how we manage our conditions, and maybe how to deal with the symptoms.

My story is one of how other people have lived with my symptoms. A story I've come to see as rare. My story is rare, because although I was lucky enough to find a community that helped me find healing, which helped me become stronger and feel accepted just as I am, I'm very aware that for many people living with mental illness, this isn't the case. For many others, in church settings they only find judgment and condemnation instead of love and acceptance.

I'm pretty sure the major cause of my mental illness was a significant trauma I experienced between the ages of eight and twenty-three, involving a parent's alcoholism, domestic violence, neglect, and ultimately, the tragic early loss of a parent. A perfect storm.

I treated the external symptoms for years, but it's only in the last eighteen months that I have finally begun to confront the deeper trauma inside of me—the core mental and psychological damage this trauma inflicted on me.

I have several mental health challenges. I have anxiety, I can have very depressive moods, and I'm a highly sensitive person (HSP). I also have PTSD caused by the trauma I mentioned above and may be very high functioning on the autistic spectrum. I identify with the autism spectrum because I get frustrated and uncomfortable when plans I've made get changed at the last minute, or I don't feel in control of things, and I have had to teach myself to pick up social cues—they don't come naturally to me.

If you met me, you probably wouldn't notice this on the surface. I'm quite high functioning and have learned to manage my mental illnesses very well. But they're still there.

Many of you feel familiar enough with anxiety and depression—our culture has become all too familiar with these in recent years. The same could be said of autism, though there are still misconceptions around this mental health condition.

Highly sensitive people are not so well understood. Many have never even heard of this condition. Being highly sensitive isn't a choice. It's not attention-seeking or making drama out of nothing or not having a thick skin. It's a neurological condition which affects twenty percent of people in the world today.

In short, HSPs bruise more easily. We can be at a party, having fun, laughing away—then someone will say something that crosses a boundary in our soul. I might know the person is joking and even think it's funny. But my brain, my emotions, will be reacting differently. I could be deeply hurt. When this happens with me,

I feel violated, personally attacked, hurt, taken advantage of. This is all going on in my brain and in my heart.

When you're in a big church community, that's not easy. In fact, it can be very uncomfortable—especially when you're having to guess at social cues all the time.

And it's with this background in mind that I share my story with you.

And although it's happened in the full glare of a home group linked to my church, I've never felt safer as part of that community. In fact, it was because of the grace, understanding, compassion, and care of my church that I've come so far.

In October 2017, I'd been dealing with my past for about a year or so. I'd worked through a lot of forgiveness and gotten lots of healing. But I was about to have the most severe depressive episode and attack of anxiety I've ever had in my life.

I'd been out of full-time work for a year, and despite hundreds of job applications, dozens of job interviews where I'd be the second or third choice, I just couldn't find permanent employment. I was out of money, and it was coming to the time where my future would no longer be in my control. I was looking at having to sell my flat, or at least rent it out whilst sleeping on someone's couch.

I remember sitting on my sofa in my warm home. The room was silent. It was just me. Silent. Without even a thought in my head. No sign of hope. Overwhelmed, alone, forgotten. I slipped off the front of the sofa and my knees went to the floor. I had no energy to even try to resist.

My vision was skewered with the depths of my tears. I had nothing left. No energy to pray. No energy to fight. Nothing to give. I had been stripped down to nothing.

I went and lay on my bed and tried to pray. And it crossed my mind right then, almost instinctively, how I might theoretically take my life.

Jump in front of a car, maybe. I even envisioned it. Almost like watching myself in a movie, I saw it in my mind, me jumping in front of a car.

I never got to the stages of planning to take my life, or making that decision. But I was on my way.

I just found the energy to message a couple of friends from church, telling them how I felt. It was all I had left.

I heard nothing for what seemed like hours. In reality, it was probably only half an hour later that I got a couple of messages. We arranged to go out for a drink to honestly discuss the situation, to get real about what was happening.

As I sat with the friends from my church, baring my soul, my anxiety, my fear to them, I felt no shame. No guilt. No fear. There was no shaming, no treating me as deficient for my anxiety, my depression, and for feeling as I had. No telling me there was something wrong with me for feeling as I did.

All I felt was grace, love, understanding.

When I went to my home group, to my church services, people all knew my story. They knew what had happened. They knew my anxiety. But they treated me without pity. They didn't patronize, or tell me I had a demon, or that I was in trouble with God because I had a mental illness.

They loved me. They accepted me. Just as I am.

Exactly as Christ loves and accepts each of us.

That week, I got the permanent job I have now. Of course, while the pressure was off, that didn't take away my anxiety.

Because mental illness doesn't go away; you just learn to manage it.

I still have recurring panic attacks, anxiety attacks, and depressive moods. I still have to manage being highly sensitive. It's still an effort to pick up social cues.

But every time I've shared these challenges with my church community, it's the same unconditional love and acceptance I find in response.

I've often felt inferior, inadequate, deficient, immature, for having mental illness. I felt fear and shame about telling people. But once I told them, that disappeared—because their response was not one of judgment, condemnation, and ignorance. No, I always felt nothing but love, grace, acceptance and understanding.

One of the major misunderstandings of mental illness, is that some people believe it's something to be fixed. That somehow those who have mental illness are deficient, less valuable, less than whole, or need to be "cured" somehow.

And of course, this is even more prevalent in religious communities.

How a church community engages with its members who have mental illnesses is important. Indeed, the Christian church should be leading the way in advocating for and supporting those with mental illness. In the church, the mentally ill should be treated with love, respect, and as equals, while also having grace and understanding our unique characteristics and challenges.

Many churches don't do this, sadly. I know people who've been driven away from church, and whose lives have had tragic consequences as a result, because they've felt alone, abandoned, and rejected by the God who, in truth, loves them unconditionally.

I've been truly blessed to be part of a different kind of community. A community of grace, love, acceptance, understanding. A community which takes me just as I am. A space I feel welcome, loved, and accepted. And a space which reminds me of the fundamental truth that God loves us all, just as we are.

My hope and prayer is that, as time passes, more churches can begin to learn how to be a safe space for those who face mental health challenges. The heart of Jesus's message is to be a welcoming space for all people to belong. A space where people know they are loved and accepted, just as they are. In so doing, the church can then become more of a reflection of Jesus and His kingdom on earth.

Depressed to Thriving—
How One Church Made a Difference

by Nancy Booth

How can the behaviors and beliefs characteristic of a particular church help a person go from a depressed state to a thriving state? The culture of my church, with its high-grace approach, the authenticity of the leaders, and the emphasis on coming alongside someone in prayer helped me do just that—moved me from depressed to thriving.

It wasn't an overnight process. And it wasn't only the church's responsibility to get me to a healthy state. Being part of the church was only one part of the holistic journey I took to get well. The church, psychotherapy, medical support, supportive family and friends, retreats, spiritual direction, and practicing self-care methods are examples of the strategies and tools I feel God provided along the journey.

However, four specific values from my church created a safe space for me during my two-year recovery process. These values allowed my health and strong faith a safe space to resurface during my journey back to wholeness.

1. No Perfect People Allowed

This value of high grace allowed me to be myself, even in my darkest moments. The church started as a small church plant. When I joined, there were about thirty attendees. I had been coming for about four years when my "dark night of the soul" hit with a vengeance.

I had been dealing with depression off and on in my midlife years. However, this particular winter hit hard. I had been working on light-box therapy for Seasonal Affective Disorder that the shorter winter days bring on. Since I had several things in place—exercise, the light box, going to bed at the right time, talk therapy—I was angry. Angry that I wasn't healed after all my hard work. Angry that I had to work so hard to be happy. Angry that it took so much work to feel even a little bit rested.

With the value of no perfect people in place, I was grateful, though, that I could walk into church without a smile on my face. I could be authentic. I could cry and sniffle. I didn't have to pretend I was in a good spot. I also didn't have to isolate myself—which is hard to do anyway in a group of thirty people.

I kept coming back because I needed the realness of the people around me and their faith. I could lean into their warmth and faith. This was especially true when I was wondering where God was in the darkness. I could ask hard questions and people didn't run away. I was not ostracized for those questions or my depression.

The church leadership remained authentic. They listened to me, prayed for me and walked alongside me. I always felt welcomed to come talk to the elders, the lead pastor, or anyone else when I felt I needed additional support. Without this authenticity and openness, my journey back toward health would have been much more difficult. Maybe I wouldn't have made it back at all.

2. WE ARE BETTER TOGETHER

I did get tired of answering the question, "How are you?" It's not that I didn't want my dear church family to care for and love me. I was bone-tired of the same answers over and over again, "Not as good as I would like." Or, "So tired." Or, "Fine," depending on who was asking.

For me, a true people-pleaser, I wanted to answer fine. I wanted the sadness, the tiredness, the feeling of wanting to run away to be done. In many ways, I didn't want to face how I was feeling, so saying fine was an avoidance tactic on my part as well. It was easier to fake it than to tell someone the truth of how I was feeling—until it wasn't easier.

The load at times would get too heavy to bear from smiling falsely. Then I would need to find someone I could really tell how I was feeling. I'm grateful that one of the elders consistently asked me, "How are you?" In some ways, I dreaded telling him I wasn't fine. However, I knew that he wanted the truth and I could be transparent with him.

Later, I asked him how that season was for him, when I repeatedly said I was *not* fine. He said he would pray for me at the moment, as well as later. He knew he couldn't fix it, but God could be involved.

My elder knew to be persistent in prayer and felt my faith would be part of the healing equation. He felt there would be a God story in the end. I am grateful for his faith that carried me when I couldn't carry myself.

After one particular trying time, I approached one of the pastors who I knew had dealt with depression. I was especially glad for his authenticity and transparency. It helped me know I was not alone and who I might approach. When talking to my pastor and telling him of my suicidal thoughts, he made me promise to "not do anything stupid," which for me was startling, like a bucket of cold water in my face.

He then proceeded to give me a word picture to which I could hold. He described a polar bear climbing a mountain in a snow storm, one step at a time. That visual resonated for me. As I reflect back now, I think the visual helped me know to take one step at a time and feel like I was being listened to that day, regardless of how hard life was at the moment. It would get better.

3. Helping People Connect and Reconnect with God

I had been serving the church in a variety of leadership capacities when the depressive episode hit. I was encouraged to take care of myself, rest, and get well. I never felt stigmatized because of my illness. I truly did need to focus on self-care to get myself back on track.

Part of that self-care meant reconnecting with God in a way I had not known before. Silence and solitude are difficult if you are too busy. Getting the help I needed from counseling, rest, and silent retreats all took time and introspection. I was freed from the leadership at church to turn inward so that I could do the healing work required.

Notice I said I was freed. I was never required, shamed, isolated, told I "should," or rejected. I felt only encouraged and lovingly held so I could see what I needed to do to get healthier.

I found resting and self-care to be quite a challenge. I knew I needed to take care of myself—eat right, exercise, go to bed at a particular time, rest. However, when I was so tired and even my thinking was not straight, caring for myself was the last thing on my mind. People continued to make sure I got to church, checked in on me when I was at church, and checked on me when I wasn't at church.

I felt loved and well-cared-for, even when I was having difficulty doing that for myself.

4. GROWING PEOPLE CHANGE

As I proceeded to work on getting better, the church continued to feed my soul through the focus on God's word, connection with other believers, and an encouragement to keep reaching out to God through prayer.

I particularly remember my pastor reminding me of 2 Peter 1:3: "His divine power has given us everything we need for a godly life through our knowledge of Him who called us by His own glory and goodness."

At the time, I was having some difficulty accessing the understanding of His divine power. Where was God when I was feeling so low? How could I access His divine power when I felt I had no power? In the end, I felt carried by His power and the prayers of my pastor and friends. It brought much hope to know that His power was there. Our discussions entailed talking and being listened to, not being preached at.

I always felt our discussions were ones where he had my heart in mind, as he lifted me up before Jesus with great grace. I left our meetings with much gratitude and great hope.

In hindsight, though, I never felt that I had to "have more faith," or "pray harder." The divine power I received was the discernment, wisdom, and guidance to access the strategies and tools I needed to get healthy again. I felt God directing me in each step of my growth and connecting me with the right people at exactly the right time.

And today?

I can report that I am healthier now than I have been in twenty years. I do the work, though. I get up in the morning for prayers and meditation, eat healthy food, pray as I go throughout the day, and take my medications as prescribed. I look to God to do the rest.

Do I still get depressive episodes? Yes, briefly, yet I know more of what to do, who to give my issues to, and where my supports are—my loving family and church family. I find that when the fear starts to rise a little about depression coming back, I take my feelings and thoughts to God, first. Then I check in on what self-care I have been doing. The last step includes how much energy I've been expending and asking myself, "What is mine to do?"

Am I back in a leadership role? Yes, I lead our prayer and care ministry now as we watch for more of God's fingerprints across our members' lives.

Is the thriving support consistent throughout the church, especially as it has grown to a church of 120? Perhaps not as it could be. The grace-filled church culture is there, yet it is difficult for everyone to reach out and grab it.

"Now it's up to you. Be on your toes—both for yourselves and your congregation of sheep. The Holy Spirit has put you in charge of these people—God's people they are—to guard and protect them. God himself thought they were worth dying for." (Acts 20:28 MSG)

The culture is in place. We want to be on our toes. The next steps may be to help all of us become more aware as we welcome those with mental health issues.

What about you and your church? What values are in place for grace, authenticity, walking alongside one another, and growing closer to God? Helping create a safe space for everyone is a big step. With prayer and intentions, you can create a thriving space for those who desire better mental health. Isn't that most of us, at one time or another?

Dragon Fighters

by TJ Atlee

The paint had worn off parts of the old floor planks, exposing the raw woodgrain. It seemed an apt metaphor as I studied the floor I sat on. The careful façade I'd built had worn thin, and I felt exposed in places that I most wanted to stay hidden.

"I can't do this. I don't *want* to do this anymore."

I briefly thought of calling someone and asking for help. All of the times that I'd reached out in the past scrolled through my mind, reminding me of why I couldn't. I would be asked what I could possibly have to be depressed about. My struggles would be dismissed. Words spoken years ago by a relative that I'd dared trust with my secret haunted me: "Christians don't get depressed, not if they're really saved. If you're depressed, it's a sign that you don't have enough faith."

I couldn't ask for help again.

I heard the muffled sounds of the movie my kids watched through the closed door. Why couldn't I breathe? Hiding in my bedroom, I hugged my knees tighter to my chest and choked out the only prayer that I could come up with, "Oh God, help me."

I'd spent the last week taking my kids to a local museum, out for ice cream, and on other little adventures. I plastered on as bright a smile as I could manage and included myself in the group photos I posted on social media. There were likes and comments about how much fun we must be having, and how I was a good mom for spending time making memories with my kids. No one knew the battle I fought behind the scenes. They couldn't know.

Christian, homeschooling moms aren't supposed to fight dragons like depression or anxiety. We're not supposed to wake up every morning fighting back tears because we don't know how to get through another day. When we say, "Stop the world, I want to get off!" we're not supposed to mean that we actually wish we could quit life. That's not the sort of thing that good moms go through.

And so I sat, huddled on the floor, listening to the dragon speak lies.

"You know, everyone would be better off without you. Think of everything they could do and accomplish if they didn't have to deal with you and your stupid problems!"

Convinced that the dragon was right, I listened to and believed more lies.

"If you were ever really honest with anyone—ever told them the real truth—you'd lose everything. No one would ever trust children to a mother like you. Everyone would be disappointed by how weak you are. No one would really care about you, they'd just feel sorry for you. You would lose *everything*."

Much as I wanted to, I couldn't just give up. My husband was still overseas on a business trip, and my kids still needed someone to take care of them. Maybe it wasn't the best reason not to give up, but it was a reason. That afternoon, it was enough. I pulled myself together enough to pretend that I was only tired when my kids asked me why I was in my room in the middle of the day. Somehow, I made it through the rest of that day until I put the kids to bed.

I sat at my desk that evening while the kids slept. If I wasn't giving up, that meant I'd have to figure out how to fight this dragon. I wrote in my journal, "Lord, will I be fighting my dragon until Heaven? If so, give me the strength to keep going. I sure don't have it within myself."

I decided to create a daily checklist of what I could do to fight this dragon, all the small things that had helped me in the past when things got dark. Exercising, journaling, taking my supplements, eating something healthy, and copying Scripture verses into my journal—all had a place on my daily list. I started calling myself a dragon fighter, hoping it would make me feel brave. Some days, I did feel brave, or at least brave enough to fight.

I still needed a lifeline of sorts; something that I could hold onto when the dragon whispered lies to me. None of the positive thinking mantras suggested by Dr. Google for fighting depression were enough. Then I found 2 Corinthians 4:16: "Therefore we do not give up. Even though our outer person is being destroyed, our inner person is being renewed day by day."

We do not give up.

Words lifted right out of scripture became my mantra, my saving grace. That day, I wrote this in my journal:

"Oh, Lord. I feel like my outer person is being destroyed! I feel like all of me is! But, I do not give up. My inner person is daily renewed—by You. Help me to remember this. Especially when my dragon returns, seeking to tear me apart. Renew me and strengthen me so I won't give up."

I wrote that verse on a sticky note and posted it by my desk. I kept journaling, even when I was frustrated, angry, and wanted to give up my fight. If I was going to be fighting dragons for the rest of my life, then I had to be honest about it somewhere, even if it was only in my journals.

Over the course of the summer, the fight slowly got easier. The dragon seemed less fierce than before, and I felt stronger and braver. I thought that maybe I had this dragon-fighting thing figured out at last.

I wish I could tell you that my story of fighting the dark dragons of mental illness included victory over them instead of what was to come. Dragons are persistent though, and they tend to hunt in packs. There are often more of them lurking in the shadows than we realize.

A troubling memory from my teen years that I'd largely ignored, refused to be ignored any longer. My dad had cornered me between the sideboard and the stove in our kitchen, looked down my shirt, and teased me about my developing figure. He thought it was a funny joke, and I didn't even realize at the time that there was anything particularly wrong with what he'd done. Because of that, I'd always felt guilty for how upset I was over it, and I did my best to bury the memories. The scene had played out on more than one occasion, but it was that particular time in the kitchen that haunted me. And in that memory, the dragons found a new way to attack.

I'd always loved the riot of color found in the changing autumn leaves. I hoped that a walk would take my mind off the troubling memories, but it turns out that you can't outrun your memories. My knees started to shake with the beginnings of a panic attack and I sat on the ground next to the dirt road. I couldn't get enough air into my lungs. Sharp pain bloomed in my chest, and my stomach churned. I wrapped my arms tightly around my midsection and repeated over and over, "He's not here. You're safe. It's okay. You're safe."

Two decades later, all of the shame, anger, fear, helplessness, and guilt came rushing back in. The most ordinary thing would bring the memory and intense emotions to the surface, and I felt like I was reliving it all over again. The resulting panic attacks were some of the worst I'd ever experienced.

The dragons were back.

Suddenly, I was back to full-blown depression and anxiety combined with the emotional fallout of dealing with my traumatic memories. Sleep eluded me most of the night, and when I did finally manage to fall asleep, nightmares tormented me. The mood swings were sudden and dramatic. I'd never felt so out-of-control in my life. I was so worn out that I relied too much on sugar and caffeine just to get through the day.

The dragons whispered their lies to me again. "Is this what it's like to finally lose your mind? Other people have been through so much worse and are just fine. Am I going crazy?" I thought maybe I was.

Out of sheer desperation, I looked up resources for Christians who were dealing with traumatic childhood memories. I found almost nothing on the topic, so I started looking up secular books, articles, and lectures.

I read about how childhood trauma affects neurodevelopment. I watched lectures given by people who had survived their own childhood traumas. I gleaned what I could from any resource and started to understand a little better exactly what was happening to me. Somehow, these people had figured out how to live with what they had endured. Maybe there was hope for me too.

I realized what I was going through was serious. During a phone call with a friend, I finally worked up the courage to admit it. My hands shook the whole time. Despite my shaking hands and the tears streaming down my face, there was some amount of relief in saying it aloud.

"I'm not okay."

It was in my old high school tutor that I found a safe person to open up to. During my teen years, she was a friend and mentor, and now she was the one on the other end of the phone when I finally admitted that something was wrong. She listened, prayed with me, and continued to be my friend.

The dragons had knocked me to the ground, but I was ready to start fighting again. Deep breath. Pick up the sword. We do not give up.

If my earlier journaling felt brutally honest, it became even more so as I processed the overwhelming emotions associated with my memories. Writing my prayers allowed me to express the hurt, frustration, and anger, and ask God to help me sort through all of the feelings and memories I didn't know how to handle.

Gradually, those open wounds started to heal a bit. The panic attacks lessened in intensity and eventually became a rare occurrence instead of a daily one. I had nights when I slept free of nightmares. I started to feel less like I was going crazy, and more like myself again.

I'm still a work in progress, and I will be one for the rest of my life. There are yet battles for me to fight this side of eternity. When the dragons return to fight, I'll hold tight to those words from 2 Corinthians and pray for the grace and strength to pick up my sword as often as I must.

Mental illness is more than any of us can handle on our own, but we aren't alone. God is with us. Always. When the dragons whisper their lies and try to convince us that we are the only one who struggles so, we combat that lie with a truth: There are a host of others who silently battle their own dragons. By the grace of God, and through the power of Christ crucified and risen, these dragons will not win. Not in the end. Until the day the dragons are defeated at last, we fight for our lives. We are not alone, and we do not give up.

SMILING AT THE WRONG STORY

BY KATIE PHILLIPS

She brings smiles wherever she goes, our little sunshine.

She has my blond hair, my mom's and my ski-slope nose, the square Hildebrand chin. When my mom and I go to the grocery store or church, even strangers wave at us, smiling at three generations out for a girls' day.

Smiling at the story they think they know.

But the real-life story is very different. The real-life story is that our little sunshine is actually my youngest cousin. The real-life story is that our sunshine's mama has been battling depression for the last three years, to the point that our sunshine has spent most of her almost-four years living with my parents. The real-life story is that my parents have exchanged their cozy empty-nester season for blocks on the floor, nap-time meltdowns, and alphabet magnets covering the fridge.

The real-life story is that two years ago today my aunt tried to take her own life.

———————

Eleven a.m. on a Friday morning. My phone rang, and I picked up. It was my oldest cousin.

"Please pray," she said, bravely fighting back sobs. "Mom shot herself."

She called EMS. She called her dad, who drives trucks and was several hours away. Then she called me.

There are no words to help in that moment, that will reassure a frightened girl and soothe away the terror and pain of betrayal and the real-life possibility that she might see her mom die.

"I'm here." On the other end of the line, I hear her talking to her mom, trying to keep her alert. In another part of the house, her sister ushered their four other siblings out the door to the neighbors'.

"I'm praying."

I couldn't help but wonder where God was in the midst of this horrifying tragedy.

"I have to go," the oldest daughter said. "The police are here."

As I packed an overnight bag, went downstairs to tell my roommate and best friend, and we hurried out to the car together, I still prayed. And wondered.

I drove long, winding roads past wheat fields lying barren under winter frost, driving to go hug on the kids who had just saved their mother's life. And I prayed. And wondered.

What was God doing in this tragedy? In some ways, I'm still wondering. In other ways, I know.

God moved the EMS to choose to do training exercises that day only five minutes from my aunt and uncle's rural farmhouse, instead of their usual location 30–45 minutes away.

God moved the hands of the paramedics and pilot rushing her to a hospital several hours away.

God moved to give me the strength to hold frightened kiddos tight and watch *The Muppets* with them while they waited for news.

God moved in the hearts of friends and strangers who gave generously when my aunt and uncle's Christian insurance organization refused to help with medical bills because the wounds were self-inflicted.

God moved to connect people to give Janice a local house to stay in when she was released from the hospital.

God moved to give us all a blessing in an eight-month reprieve last year, to remind us of the beautiful, vibrant person trapped inside the shell of depression.

God moved.

———————

That day two years ago was far from my first encounter with depression and mental illness, though it was the most severe.

As a child, and again in high school, my strong, chill, always-positive mother went through seasons of severe anxiety and panic attacks. During a tear-filled attack, I would run a hot bath, rub her back, and sing the old song she taught me as a child—

God will make a way, when there seems to be no way.
He works in ways we cannot see.
He will make a way for me.
He will be my guide, hold me closely to His side.
With love and strength, for each new day.
He will make a way.

A *Wonder Woman* movie poster hangs on the wall of my sister's bedroom. For some, it represents entertainment or a nerdy bent. For her, it represents who she is in her battle with depression. For her—for us—it represents that she lives, loves others, and she is therefore strong and victorious.

In college, I walked the sidewalks of campus many late nights with my sister, encouraging her through her own battles with anxiety and depression. The struggle has carried on over the years. The conversations, the texts speaking words you never want anyone to say about themselves, let alone your beloved older sister.

The days when depression and anxiety spoke, lashing out with hurtful words, instead of the kind, compassionate woman I know her to be.

A few years ago, in a bedroom far away across the sea, I spoke to my brother over Skype, speaking encouraging words into his heart that never seemed to penetrate his deep depression.

He'd graduated with a degree in agricultural economics in the midst of economic repression, lived at home for over a year looking for work, and found himself living with severe knee pain when he did finally get a job a local factory. On good days, he'd sit at the supper table and entertain us all with his dry wit. On bad days, he came home from work and went straight to his room. Sometimes he'd call me to talk. Those were hard days. Sometimes he wouldn't talk at all. Those days were even harder.

————————————

They say it's good to talk about your struggles, and usually that's true. But I find I don't talk about this struggle very much.

How do we talk about mental health? How do you begin this difficult conversation?

In the church, most people say those who struggle with anxiety and depression just need to pray and trust God more. And that may be true, in part. But it's not the whole truth, which makes it even more dangerous than an outright lie.

In the secular world, most people say depression and anxiety are a result of an imbalance in brain chemistry or a result of past trauma. That's often true too. But it's not the whole truth.

We can't even begin to understand the complexities of how our brains work. How can we hope to understand mental illness with such simplistic explanations?

It's trauma—and so much more. It's a brain chemistry imbalance—and so much more. It's spiritual attack and conflict—and yet more.

And somewhere in our obsession with finding the cause, with "fixing" the problem, we lose sight of the person. The people, for we all suffer *as a result of* mental illness, even if we don't struggle with it directly. This is my story—battling with and against the wounds from those I love the most.

We punish the person for a moment of weakness when we should be picking them up and nursing their wounds and showing compassion to their family.

We say silly but hurtful things like, "Have you tried thinking positive thoughts?" to someone who battles every day to find the emotional fortitude to get up, to care for children, to go to work. They're trying, or they wouldn't still be here. Still be fighting.

Or, we don't say anything at all, because we don't know what to say.

Sometimes, that's best. Sometimes, that person just needs a friend to sit with them in the dark, to hold their hand and silently remind them that they are loved and never alone. Sometimes, more is needed, and we don't know what that more is, so we deal with our own sense of shame and failure for not being enough.

Some of these family members are in a good season, and for that I'm so thankful.

My brother has made wonderful friends, is living with some Christian guys, helped his team win their ultimate frisbee league—thanks to quitting his job to have knee surgery—and is now working full-time with a carpenter finishing high-end houses.

We are enjoying a season of reprieve with my sister the last few months, and the ever-more-frequent glimpses of the sister I knew growing up makes the occasional tough day easier to stomach.

Other family members' stories and seasons are made ever more difficult by the relentless progression of time without visible healing.

But still, we keep on.

We read storybooks to our sunshine before bed and celebrate her first letters. We enjoy the bright days, embracing every moment, and cling to God in the hard days.

We pray. We wonder.

We wait.

HEADS I WIN, TAILS YOU LOSE

BY VIRGINIA PILLARS

Acceptance. Rejection. I don't know what I'd yell if I tossed a coin in the air with these words on it instead of the ones we carry in our pockets. I know that I have a fifty-fifty chance for either reaction with mental illness.

Rejection or acceptance, or another way to think about it, stigma or understanding. Our family experienced both as we dealt with the challenges that came with our daughter's diagnosis of schizophrenia. Acceptance, she won. Rejection, she lost. We learned about the wildly different reactions of church staff members and congregations during our crash course on mental illness.

Up until 2004, I lived in a naïve world. I thought I understood mental illness. Sure, I knew about it and could name a few people that I knew who dealt with different illnesses. In reality, I didn't have a clue. In my inexperienced microcosm, I also thought I could turn to the church community for support during a mental health crisis. I discovered that, in some cases, I could, but not always. That proverbial coin landed on both sides as we encountered contradictory reactions when mental illness invaded our family.

In 2004, our twenty-four-year-old daughter, Amber, took a job as a youth minister in a large church. With a college degree in hand, it seemed like the perfect fit for her, and she gave it her all. She loved the Lord and wanted to share her enthusiasm for faith with young people. She and a coworker implemented a youth program for grades seven through twelve. Since I had known the pastor of the congregation for many years, I felt that she hit the jackpot when she moved about an hour away from her childhood home where she grew up with her dad, Roy, her three brothers, and me.

My first lesson on the reality of church support with mental illnesses happened during Amber's psychotic break, which occurred during her time there.

Before I flip the coin and call out the results, I want to point out that the office manager went out on a limb when she called to me to express her concern about Amber's odd behavior. In her view, this was a big change in Amber. She didn't know how I'd react, but she reached out anyway. Her phone call alerted me that something was terribly wrong, and for that, I'll always feel grateful.

The first coin flip landed on tails.

After a conversation with Amber, I jumped into my car and drove ninety miles an hour to get to her. During that drive, my mind assaulted me with "What if?" and "Is she suicidal?" That hour drive seemed to take forever. On December 9, 2004, I brought Amber home with me for what I thought was a three-day weekend of rest. Instead, it morphed into four years.

That night, as I drove home with her, I suggested a doctor visit and she agreed. The doctor who met with us the next day diagnosed her with depression and prescribed an antidepressant plus a one-week work release. Reluctantly, Amber agreed to the medication and we called her office manager before we faxed the release.

With Amber's permission, I listened to the amicable conversation between them. "Rest up and come back when you feel better," Judith, the office manager said to her. Just what I'd hoped to hear—encouragement and understanding.

One week passed and the work release expired, but the invisible hold on Amber's mind tightened its grip. Her paranoia became visible to us. Within days, she became convinced that television programs, newspaper and magazine articles were all about her and her life as part of a conspiracy against her. Roy and I tried to talk her out of this in our uneducated efforts to make sense of it all. We soon learned that we had wasted our breath. No amount of explanation changed her trapped mind. We knew she couldn't go back to work for at least a few weeks.

I contacted Judith and the pastor. I explained that the medicine might take weeks to bring improvement and Amber needed more time off. Again, I heard compassion and understanding from both. "Just keep in touch, let us know how she does. She has our prayers."

Later, Judith called Amber's cell phone. I leaned my head close to Amber's while she held the phone at an angle so we could both hear. I kept silent as I let Amber talk.

I tasted stigma for the first time that day. I wanted to spit out the bitterness. Judith didn't sound like the same woman I had spoken with earlier. She began with, "When will you come back to work?" When Amber couldn't give her an answer, she berated her, "We have to know. You have to give me a date," she demanded.

Amber's mannerisms and facial expressions screamed, "I can't handle this!" as I witnessed her anxiety level rise. I shook my head and mouthed, "Tell her you have to go."

Amber ended the call.

"Don't listen to her," I said. "Just concentrate on your health. I'll talk to her from now on."

During the next few weeks, as Amber slipped out of the world I knew into a world I couldn't reach, I kept the pastor and Judith informed. During this time, she checked herself into a local hospital, but left AMA (against medical advice). Within a few weeks, we forced her into hospitalization through a court committal.

Again, inexperienced me thought she'd improve once she received the antipsychotic medication through an injection under a doctor's care in the hospital. My hopes sank as I watched her spiral downward until she lived in a world without language. She stared into space most of the time with only seconds of coherency before she retreated to a different reality.

As we prepared to transfer her to a different hospital, I spoke with the pastor. During the phone call I explained the extent of her illness, our heartache with the uncertainty of the length of time she needed to stay in a hospital setting, and the fact that we didn't have a diagnosis yet. "I don't think she'll come back to work for months," I relayed to him.

He sounded concerned and reminded me of their prayers for her. "We'll look for a long-term sub and keep her on the insurance plan until her contract expires in June," he assured me.

That conversation filled me with hope. I felt like they had our backs as we transferred Amber to the third hospital in less than a month.

Until the letter arrived from Judith.

"Dear Amber,

This letter is to inform you that due to your inability to effectively perform the job...and not

returning to work after your doctor's certificate
expired...we consider this your voluntary resignation effective immediately.

I know we discussed that we would pay your
health insurance..."

The letter went on to explain that they wouldn't pay for it as
promised, but she could buy it through a temporary insurance
company. It ended with keep in touch and you are in our prayers.

I felt as if they'd kicked me in the gut. No job, no insurance.
Pay for it herself? With what? I wanted to scream at them. *She's in
the hospital for who knows how long! Thanks for showing us Christ's
love and compassion!* Anger boiled over in me as I swallowed the
bitter dose of rejection. *Keep in touch? Yeah, right! Would you do
this if she had cancer?*

We broke all communication with them.

The lack of insurance threw Amber into the world of social
services. As an adult with no insurance, she had zero means to
pay the hospitals and doctors or buy the much-needed medication. By now, all the money she had worked hard to save had
already gone to pay her bills. We applied for conservatorship and
guardianship so we could handle all her legal affairs. We knew
her state-of-mind couldn't handle even the smallest decision, let
alone the mountain of paperwork she faced.

"How do people without family get all this done?" I asked
myself. *No wonder the mentally ill end up homeless on the street.*

Flip the coin. Heads, she wins.

We did receive support. Amber's best friend, Brooke demonstrated to us what love in action can look like. I started to call
her an example of *God with skin*. She illustrated Christian love

and compassion from the very beginning and restored my faith in people.

On December 9, after that first phone call from Judith as I drove in a panic to Amber, I called Brooke. "Keep Amber on the line until I get there," I begged. When I arrived at Amber's apartment, she had her cell phone to her ear as she chatted with Brooke. Relief overrode fear for a few minutes.

Brooke continued to live her call to action when she dropped everything to rush to Amber's side every time she knew there was a need. Our son Mitchell pointed Roy and me in the direction of the local National Alliance on Mental Illness (NAMI) and we learned about Hope for Tomorrow, a class that they offered for parents with children affected by mental illness. Even though Amber wasn't a child, the director of the local chapter encouraged us to attend. "You can benefit from the lessons." We both wanted to attend to learn about this monster that had invaded our family, but we didn't want to leave Amber home alone. Not even for a few hours. I called Brooke.

"I usually have Bible study that night, but I'll come over to hang out with Amber instead," she promised.

My encouragement thermometer rose a few degrees. Amber just thought her friend came to visit, not that we needed someone to stay with her. Her trust in Brooke and her dad and me remained high as the psychosis continued to slash at her mind.

Brooke continued her support of our family. After we went to court to force Amber into the hospital, Brooke rang the bell for admittance into the locked ward to see her friend. I can still see her slide through the door with a stuffed, brown puppy in her hand. She crossed the sterile room to the corner where Amber and I sat on the tiled floor below the window. Emotional pain seeped from my pores as Amber shouted obscenities at the staff. I had tried to calm her down but failed. Instead, I cringed in silence, helpless to halt the tumbled thoughts in her mind.

Brooke ignored the awful words. Instead, she snuggled beside Amber. She wrapped her arm around Amber's shoulder, "How ya doin', sweetie?"

Amber's anger dissolved as she clutched the stuffed animal to her chest and rested her head on Brooke's shoulder. The three of us stayed that way until visiting hours ended.

The NAMI class gave me the strength to share our situation with our families and closest friends. Family members stopped to see Amber at the hospital. It seemed every day she had a visitor or two. I don't think many of them had ever stepped into a locked ward before, but they saw someone in need, put aside their qualms, and spent time with her.

> "'When did we see you sick or in prison and visit you?' And the King will reply, 'Truly I tell you, whatever you did for one of the least of these brothers of mine, you did for me.'"
>
> —Matthew 25:39–40

During the NAMI class I heard a saying, "No one brings you a casserole when your family member is in the psychiatric ward at the hospital." I guess our church friends hadn't taken the course because one evening I opened the front door to see one couple in front of me with a casserole dish in hand. "I know things are rough right now. Maybe this will make today a bit easier," she said.

"Oh, thank you," I said. "Please, stay and eat with us?" I asked them.

"No, we don't want to intrude," he said in an apologetic voice.

Because my days had become a revolving door of hospitals, doctors, nursing staffs, and Amber's deteriorating mental state, I craved some normalcy. "Please, we could use the company," I begged.

With some hesitation, they joined us. That evening gave me a boost. After our meal, they sat with Roy and me as we unloaded our grief on them. They didn't say anything. They just sat and cried with us. It reminded me of the second chapter of Job when his friends came to him.

> "Then they sat down upon the ground with him
> seven days and seven nights, but none of them
> spoke a word to him; for they saw how great was
> his suffering."
>
> —Job 2:13

Our faith community that had surrounded us for most of our married life illustrated to me how to treat a family in the clutches of mental illness.

In addition to visiting Amber, cards, letters, and faxes arrived almost daily at the hospital, filled with words of encouragement to her. Some even sent small gifts for Amber—chocolates, lotions, stuffed animals—anything that might boost her spirits. We received many cards and letters too, along with promises of prayers for our family.

All of these small acts helped us to stay afloat as the hurricane-force gales of mental illness pounded us without mercy.

It helped her hospitalization feel closer to normal, more like a surgical procedure than a psychotic break. People of faith upheld us as we dealt with our world of confusion. We didn't feel alone.

After forty-two days of hospitalization that winter, Amber came home to continue her journey towards recovery that lasted for more than the next three years. Brooke stayed a constant in Amber's life. She demonstrated with love the passage in Deuteronomy 31:6: "Be strong and courageous. Do not be afraid or terrified because of them, for the Lord your God goes with you; he will never leave you nor forsake you."

Instead of running away from a scary situation, she ran to Amber with outstretched arms. At the time, Amber couldn't drive because of the sedating drugs she had to take. Brooke picked her up each week and took her to her Bible study where she introduced Amber to a close-knit group of faith-filled young professionals. People her age. People who accepted Amber for who she was that day. No judgments, no expectations, just open hearts to love.

Brooke also came on Sunday so Amber could go to the worship service with her new friends. That summer, and for the summers that followed, Amber joined them for sand volleyball and softball each week. These friendships provided an important part of the equation for her recovery. Instead of isolation—all too common with schizophrenia—she immersed herself in social settings. Amber found acceptance from her peers, something Roy and I couldn't do for her.

Once Amber felt ready to return to work part-time, the church that she'd attended with Brooke and her new friends hired her to help in the daycare program. Again, acceptance helped her move forward as she walked her journey with baby steps of improvement. After several months, the pastor asked Amber if she'd consider a video to talk about her illness and the importance of faith in the recovery process of mental illness. To my surprise, she agreed.

The day the church shared the video, Roy and I joined her at one of the services. That day, over a thousand families watched as Amber told her story. Afterward, we stood to the side in awe as her faith community surrounded her with congratulatory hugs. Amber walked out of the church that day a winner. The sweetness of acceptance dissolved any bitter taste I still had from the church that fired her.

We tossed the proverbial coin in our church, too, when we approached our pastor to share our situation. We won the toss as he gave us compassionate counseling. "God is a merciful God who loves her." He told us to call him when we needed someone to listen.

Amber returned to full-time employment in a different role in 2009, four years after her "voluntary resignation" as a youth minister. After two years, she felt called to return to youth ministry and secured a job quickly. By then, she'd stayed in recovery for over two years. At first, she thrived. She fell in love with the students and families. And they loved her. She told me about notes and emails from them during our daily phone chats. She'd overcome her illness and performed her job well. Things went well for the first few months.

In January, during a small group sharing at a retreat that she attended, she shared with her coworker some of her struggles from the past. Overnight, things changed. It seemed as if she'd tossed the coin once again and it landed on tails. Rejection began to raise its ugly head once more.

The staff started to treat her differently. They tightened control on her decisions until they micromanaged everything that she did with the youth. Through our phone conversations she shared the disapproval vibes that she felt. To her it felt like she'd lost all their trust. Still, she gave it her all. Her devotion to the youth overrode the frustration she felt.

Five and a half months after she'd started, on February 14, the pastor called her into his office and demanded her immediate resignation. She had to clean out her office that day and turn in her keys. Devastated, she called us. To add further insult, she heard later from a parent that he announced at the following Sunday service that she had resigned due to illness. Stigma reached out and slapped her across the face. Hard.

The sting from the smack lingered as she moved home, but she didn't allow it to fester. She searched for a job and, a short time later, she found one and moved on.

Since she lost two flips of the proverbial coin, she had chosen to steer clear of youth ministry. Her heart remains with youth, so she has worked with young people for the past six years. In her new position, Amber kept her secret hidden for almost a year. Only after she'd developed a deep friendship with a coworker did she share. This time when she tossed the coin, it landed on heads. Instead of stigma and rejection, she gained acceptance and admiration.

As I look back over the past thirteen years, I can ponder each situation and can find the thumbprint of God. I don't harbor bitter feelings about the faith communities who rejected her. I've realized that each one had a part of God's larger plan for her. We just couldn't see it at the time.

When she lost her job and insurance, it threw her into the social services network where she qualified for financial assistance. We learned later that because of the inequality of parity laws at that time, she'd maxed out her insurance coverage for psychiatric care at about the same time. She'd used the thirty days allowed for inpatient and psychiatric care. Had she not been forced out of her job with insurance benefits, she would've shouldered the financial responsibility for all her hospital stays, doctor and therapist appointments, and medications for the rest of the year. The debt would have followed her for the rest of her life.

The acceptance she received in the congregation she found with Brooke became an integral factor in the equation for her recovery where she's stayed since 2009. Even the second youth minister job where rejection hurt her brought her to the community where she still resides today.

Amber broke out of the prison of mental illness when schizophrenia dealt her most of the nasty symptoms it has to offer. Instead, she learned to thrive within the company of faith-filled people who clothed her with love and acceptance.

> "I needed clothes and you clothed me, I was sick
> and you looked after me, I was in prison and
> you came to visit me."
>
> —Matthew 25:36

About the Authors

Several authors have chosen to remain anonymous. There are a variety of reasons for the anonymity. Some want to protect themselves or their families, others are simply not ready to release to the world the nature of their mental illnesses, and still others have social media platforms built around pen names. Regardless of the reasons, Llama Publishing wants to honor the desire to stay anonymous. A brief bio for each person who chose not to remain anonymous is listed below.

Nancy Booth, a member of Ezra Church in Wisconsin, is a writer, life coach, and spiritual director who encourages women to find freedom as they discover who they are in God's eyes. Her coaching and writing focus on building a healthy, purposeful, peaceful mind, heart, body, and soul. She can be found at nancyboothcoaching.com.

Heather Cook is a grateful believer in Jesus Christ. In her nearly forty years, she has survived a myriad of abuses and developed post-traumatic stress disorder. After many years of carrying secrets, she faced the memories she tried to suppress, allowed herself to grieve, and sought healing from the Great Physician. She lives in beautiful middle Tennessee with her husband of eighteen years and four children.

Karen deBlieck's writing reflects the tension of identity and sense of belonging she struggled with as a black American born in Japan and adopted by white Canadian missionaries. From a young age she found solace in putting her thoughts and feelings on the page. Writing in poem, short story, and novel form, her pieces are emotionally and conflict-charged. Check out more about Karen at karendeblieck.com.

Lindsay A. Franklin is the best-selling author of *Adored: 365 Devotions for Young Women* and *The Story Peddler*, an award-winning editor, and a homeschooling mom of three. She would wear pajama pants all the time if it were socially acceptable. She lives in her native San Diego with her scruffy-looking nerf-herder husband, their precious geeklings, three demanding thunder pillows (a.k.a. cats), and a stuffed wombat with his own Instagram following. You can learn more about Lindsay at her website: lindsayafranklin.com.

Stephanie Guido has loved reading since she was four years old when her mother found her studiously examining *Little House on the Prairie* page by page and insisting she could understand every word. So, it is most fitting that she writes and edits for a living with Quill Pen Editorial, and she's now working on her own first novel as well as shorter fiction and non-fiction pieces.

Josh Hardt is a Christ-follower, avid reader, ecumenical nerd, and lover of puns. He lives in the Midwest with his wife and two high-energy children. When not living in worlds of others' devising, Josh enjoys nighttime walks and board games. He's currently hard at work on his first novel. He is also one part of the magic that happens on the Lasers, Dragons, and Keyboards podcast.

Janeen Ippolito believes words transform worlds and loves empowering people to write with excellence and boldness. She creates writing resources and writes stories about misfits who own their scars and defy the darkness. She's also an experienced teacher, editor, author coach, and the president of Uncommon Universes Press. In her spare time, she enjoys sword-fighting with her missionary husband, reading, and wood-burning. Connect with Janeen at her website: janeenippolito.com.

Joel Larson is Aurora Behavioral Health System's Manager of Chaplain Services and oversees the chaplain services for patients, consults with patients, and leads spirituality group sessions for adults and adolescents. Joel has a Masters of Divinity from Golden Gate Baptist Theological Seminary and a Masters of Arts in Human Services Counseling from Liberty University. He served as an Arizona National Guard Chaplain Assistant conducting counseling sessions and teaching suicide prevention and stress first aid techniques. Joel worked as a mobile crisis therapist and volunteered as a pastor at a local church.

Chris Morris is the founder of Llama Publishing, LLC. As a champion of indie publishing, he has published two indie books and been a contributing author to two others. Chris regularly teaches at writing conferences as a keynote and a faculty member on topics ranging from self-publishing effectively to building your writing craft with God. You can find more of his writing at chrismorriswrites.com.

Anne Peterson is a poet, speaker, and published author who is a regular contributor to Crosswalk. Anne has published fourteen books including her memoir, *Broken: A Story of Abuse, Survival and Hope*. Anne believes life is hard. She writes words to make it softer. Connect with Anne on her website annepeterson.com or find her articles on Medium.

Katie Phillips is a fiction editor and author coach helping women authorpreneurs writing sci-fi and fantasy to create breakthrough in their writing craft and career. She has experienced first-hand the effects of depression, anxiety, and other mental illnesses and is passionate about the church supporting everyone affected and helping them find hope and healing. Katie grew up a farm girl and lives with her husband in her hometown of Wichita, Kansas.

Virginia Pillars detailed her journey through mental illness with her adult child in her memoir, *Broken Brain, Fortified Faith: Lessons of Hope Through a Child's Mental Illness*, winner of the 2017 Selah Award and the CWG Seal of Approval. She contributed to *Grief Diaries Poetry, Prose & More* and *themighty.com*. Virginia speaks on mental illness and volunteers for the NAMI (National Alliance on Mental Illness) organization as an educator/support group leader. She blogs at virginiapillars.com.

James Prescott is a writer, podcaster, and mental health advocate. He is author of several books, including *Mosaic Of Grace - God's Beautiful Reshaping Of Our Broken Lives*. He also hosts the *Poema Podcast* on creativity & spirituality, and co-hosts the *Creating Normal* podcast on creativity and mental illness. Connect with James on Twitter at @JamesPrescott77 & find more of his work at jamesprescott.co.uk.

Aaron J. Smith is a father, writer, nerd, and coffee drinker. He hates writing about himself. It's the worst. He lives with Bipolar II and fiercely believes in mental health advocacy to remove stigma and shame associated with mental illness. He also likes cats. Aaron lives in the Pacific Northwest with his two kids. He has been featured on several prominent websites and published anthologies. You can find him at CulturalSavage.com and on Twitter @CulturalSavage.

30427093R00104